Free access to accompanying content on Oxfordmedicine.com/introanaesthesia

The print copy of *Introducing Anaesthesia* you have purchased comes with free access to the accompanying online video content on Oxfordmedicine.com. To view this, you will need to create an account using the access token on this card. Please use the correct URL below based on your location when registering this token.

Customers outside North and South America, please visit: **https://subscriberservices.sams.oup.com/token** to set up access.

Customers in North and South America, please visit: **https://ams.oup.com/order/OMINTANAPRDSCRIP** to set up access.

Please keep this card for future reference as, in the event of a query, you may be asked to return it. Please note that as part of the registration process you will be informed of our terms and conditions, and will be asked to accept these to confirm your online access.

unique code: AT14509412860160

The online access provided free with this book is for individuals who have purchased a personal copy only, and this will be verified as part of the access process. Users of library copies should ask their librariar about access in their institution.

Customer support

Customers outside North & South Americ
Tel: +44 (0) 1865 353705
Email: onlinesubscriptions@oup.com

Customers in North & South America
Tel: 1-800-334-4249 ext. 6484
Email: oxfordonline@oup.com

Introducing Anaesthesia

A curriculum-based guide

Introducing Anaesthesia

A curriculum-based guide

Dr Paul Greig

Clinical Research Fellow, University of Oxford, Oxford, UK

Dr Nicholas Crabtree

Consultant Anaesthetist, Nuffield Department of Anaesthetics, John Radcliffe Hospital, Oxford University Hospitals NHS Trust and Honorary Senior Clinical Lecturer, University of Oxford, Oxford, UK

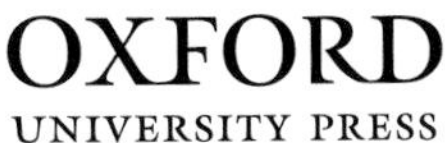

OXFORD
UNIVERSITY PRESS

Great Clarendon Street, Oxford, OX2 6DP,
United Kingdom

Oxford University Press is a department of the University of Oxford. It furthers the University's objective of excellence in research, scholarship, and education by publishing worldwide. Oxford is a registered trade mark of Oxford University Press in the UK and in certain other countries

Impression: 9 8 7 6 5 4 3 2 1

First Edition published in 2014

Published in the United States of America by Oxford University Press
198 Madison Avenue, New York, NY 10016, United States of America

British Library Cataloguing in Publication Data
Data available

Library of Congress Control Number: 2014948239

ISBN 978–0–19–871670–9

Printed in Great Britain by
Ashford Colour Press Ltd, Gosport, Hampshire

Preface

'In somno securitas'

—motto of the Association of Anaesthetists of Great Britain and Ireland

For those of you starting your career in anaesthesia, welcome to an exciting and challenging specialty. For those of you who are working in anaesthesia with a view to a career in another acute care specialty, we hope that you enjoy your time working with us and that you find the experience a useful addition to your medical training.

Anaesthesia is a specialty that has an impact on a huge number of patients. Often, people fear the anaesthetic more than the surgery. 'What if I wake up, doctor' or 'what if I don't wake up, doctor?' are commonly heard from our patients. With careful planning and sound techniques, risks from anaesthesia have been greatly reduced to the point where serious anaesthetic morbidity is a thankfully rare event.

In a practical specialty like anaesthetics there is a limit to how much can be taught from a book. The best way to learn anaesthesia is to get stuck in on the wards, in theatre, and in the simulator, but we hope that you will find this book a helpful companion as you take your first steps in our specialty.

The aim of this book is to accompany your first 3 months of anaesthesia as you learn the basics. As a syllabus, we have used the Royal College of Anaesthetists' Initial Assessment of Competency (the IAC), an assessment everyone in anaesthetics must pass before they can conduct anaesthesia without direct supervision. Reading this book will not turn you into an anaesthetist, but we hope that it will help you to make some sense of the steep learning curve that we remember going through when we started.

Anaesthesia is a challenging, technical, and frequently highly rewarding specialty. It offers a unique opportunity to witness extremes of human physiology in action and to see the effects of intervention in real time. Most importantly, there is the opportunity to make what is a stressful and difficult event for many patients a little bit easier.

Paul Greig FRCA
Nick Crabtree FRCA
October 2013

Contents

Acknowledgements

The authors wish to thank Dr Helen Higham, director of the Oxford Centre for Simulation, Training, and Research, for kind permission to use the simulation facilities in the recording of the video sequences used in this text. We are also grateful for the huge amount of support and inspiration that the staff of the Centre have offered during many years of teaching with them.

We also would like to thank Dr Claire Frampton and Miss Julie Darbyshire for their unwavering support and assistance during the development of this work, and Ms Geraldine Jeffers for helping us to navigate the shoals of manuscript preparation by making a complex process comprehensible to us.

Thanks to Dr Jo Kerr, Ms Rosie Warren, Dr Steve Webster-Edge, Mrs Kim Lovegrove, Mr Alex Rawlings, and Mr Alan Inglis for their tireless efforts in helping us to deliver the training course on which this book is based.

Finally, a big thank you to all of the trainees who have taken part in our courses. Your enthusiasm and dedication continue to amaze and inspire us.

Videos

The authors have included nine videos which demonstrate and/or explore important aspects of anaesthesia practice. Screen shots of videos are included as figures at key points in the text, and readers are directed to the online **video appendix** where appropriate. Please note this is currently not available for ebook customers until further notice.

You can access the videos here: www.oxfordmedicine.com/introanaesthesia

Videos include:

1. How to check an anaesthetic machine using the sequence taken from the *Association of Anaesthetists of Great Britain and Ireland Machine Checks* guidance document.
2. A flow chart which illustrates the various steps of a general anaesthetic and the issues which should be considered at each point.
3. *Just a routine operation: human factors in patient safety* illustrates the importance of good communication and teamwork in preventing anaesthetic disasters. Reproduced with kind permission of Martin Bromiley and the NHS Institute for Innovation and Improvement.
4. A short video sequence which illustrates a ventricular fibrillation rhythm.
5. A short video sequence which illustrates a pulseless ventricular tachycardia rhythm.
6. A short video sequence which illustrates an example of a presenting rhythm that, if it occurred during cardiac arrest, would represent pulseless electrical activity.
7. A short video sequence which illustrates asystole.
8. A short video sequence which illustrates an SBAR handover.
9. A short video demonstrates how the defibrillator marks QRS complexes after the 'sync' button has been pressed.

Symbols and abbreviations

°C	degree Celsius
CD	controlled drug
®	registered trademark
™	trademark
=	equal to
<	less than
>	more than
α	alpha
β	beta
δ	delta
κ	kappa
μ	mu
AAGBI	Association of Anaesthetists of Great Britain and Ireland
AF	atrial fibrillation
ALS	advanced life support
APL	automatic pressure-limiting (valve)
aPTT	activated partial thromboplastin time
ASA	American Society of Anesthesiologists
AV	atrioventricular
BURP	Backwards–Upwards–Rightwards–Pressure
CGO	common gas outlet
cm	centimetre
cmH_2O	centimetre of water
CNS	central nervous system
CO_2	carbon dioxide
COAD	chronic obstructive airways disease
COX	cyclo-oxygenase
CPR	cardiopulmonary resuscitation
CSF	cerebrospinal fluid
CTZ	chemoreceptor trigger zone
DAS	Difficult Airway Society
DC	direct current
DVT	deep vein thrombosis

ECG	electrocardiogram
ENT	ear, nose, and throat
$EtCO_2$	end-tidal carbon dioxide concentration
FGF	fresh gas flow
FiO_2	fractional inspired oxygen concentration
FRC	functional residual capacity
g	gram
G	gauge
GI	gastrointestinal
h	hour
HME	heat and moisture exchange
Hz	hertz
ICP	intracranial pressure
ICU	intensive care unit
IM	intramuscular
INR	international normalized ratio
ITU	intensive therapy unit
IV	intravenous
kg	kilogram
kPa	kilopascal
L	litre
LA	local anaesthetic
LMA	laryngeal mask airway
LMWH	low-molecular-weight heparin
m	metre
MAC	minimum alveolar concentration
MAO-I	monoamine oxidase-inhibitor
MAP	mean arterial pressure
mg	milligram
MH	malignant hyperthermia
min	minute
mL	millilitre
mm	millimetre
mmHg	millimetre of mercury
mmol	millimole
mV	millivolt
NAPQI	N-acetyl-p-benzo-quinoneimine

NCEPOD	National Confidential Enquiry into Patient Outcome and Death
NG	nasogastric
NIBP	non-invasive blood pressure
NICE	National Institute for Health and Clinical Excellence
NIST	non-interchangeable screw thread
nm	nanometre
NSAID	non-steroidal anti-inflammatory drug
ODP	operating department practitioner
Pa	pascal
PCA	patient-controlled analgesia
PCEA	patient-controlled epidural analgesia
pCO_2	partial pressure of carbon dioxide
PDPH	post-dural puncture headache
PEEP	positive end-expiratory pressure
PONV	post-operative nausea and vomiting
PR	per rectum
PRN	pro re nata (as required)
PT	prothrombin time
qds	quarter die sumendus (four times daily)
RSI	rapid sequence induction
s	second
SpO_2	saturation of oxygen
SVT	supraventricular tachycardia
TCI	target-controlled infusion
TIVA	total intravenous anaesthesia
UK	United Kingdom
VF	ventricular fibrillation
VIE	vacuum-insulated evaporator
V/Q	ventilation/perfusion
VT	ventricular tachycardia
WHO	World Health Organization

Chapter 1

Anaesthetic equipment

1.1 Introduction

The safe practice of anaesthesia requires familiarity with a wide range of equipment. The anaesthetist should be ready to use any of the following equipment and must have detailed knowledge of its operation.

1.2 The anaesthetic machine

The anaesthetic machine is one of the most important pieces of equipment and is fundamental to delivering safe anaesthesia. It can seem like a complex and intimidating device to use, but fundamentally it is designed to fulfil only one purpose: to take a variety of medical gases and mix them in a manner specified by the anaesthetist, before delivering them in a controlled way to the patient.

1.2.1 Piped medical gases

Most anaesthetic machines will take their primary gas supply from the hospital pipeline supply. Some theatres, particularly those separate from the hospital's main theatre block, may only have cylinder supplies.

Pipeline supplies have the advantage that they draw their gases from a central location in the hospital and should therefore never run out!

There are three gases commonly supplied to theatres via pipeline: oxygen, medical air, and nitrous oxide. Medical vacuum is also commonly taken from a pipeline supply. Although not a gas per se, the principles of its delivery and connection to the anaesthetic machine are similar.

Each gas is supplied to an outlet found either in the wall of theatre or from a pendant hanging from the roof. These outlets are called Schrader valves. The valves are colour-coded, and each outlet is of a slightly different size and shape, so it should not be possible to misconnect hoses in theatre.

Hoses take the gases from the outlet to the anaesthetic machine. Each hose is also colour-coded, and they connect to the back of the anaesthetic machine via a screw connection. These connections are unique to each gas (termed a non-interchangeable screw thread, NIST) and are designed to minimize the risk of misconnection at the machine end. These connections are seen in Fig 1.1.

1.2.1.1 *Oxygen*

- **Schrader valve colour:** white
- **Hose colour:** white
- **Supply pressure:** 400 kPa.

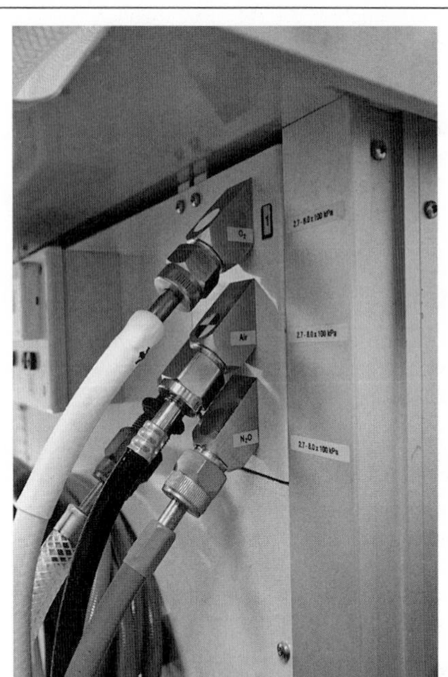

Fig 1.1 This image illustrates the pipeline connections at the back of an anaesthetic machine. Note the three hoses are colour-coded: oxygen is white, air is black, and nitrous oxide is blue. The pipelines are coupled to the machine at an NIST connector.

Oxygen is supplied to the pipeline system either from a vacuum-insulated evaporator (VIE), a cylinder manifold, or from an oxygen concentrator.

A VIE is a large tank, rather similar in principle to a Thermos® flask, which stores liquid oxygen at low temperatures. When oxygen is required the liquid in the VIE is allowed to warm and evaporate, and the resulting gas is passed to the hospital pipeline.

A cylinder manifold is simply a bank of very large cylinders (much larger than those found on the anaesthetic machine) that supply their contents to the whole hospital.

An oxygen concentrator is typically used in remote or temporary hospitals where a regular supply would be impractical. It draws in atmospheric air and processes it, delivering oxygen with a concentration of around 95% to the hospital supply.

1.2.1.2 *Medical air*

- **Schrader valve colour:** black and white
- **Hose colour:** black
- **Supply pressure:** 400 kPa (for anaesthetic machine connection) or 700 kPa (to drive pneumatic surgical tools).

A cylinder manifold can supply medical air in a manner similar to that described for oxygen, or air can be drawn from a compressor.

A compressor is a device that takes filtered atmospheric air and raises its pressure to that of the hospital pipeline supply.

Note that medical air is supplied at two different pressures in theatre: 400 kPa for connection to the anaesthetic machine, and 700 kPa used to drive pneumatic surgical tools. The connections for each pressure are labelled on the Schrader valve, and the valves themselves differ in shape and size to prevent misconnection. The colour coding for each is the same.

1.2.1.3 *Nitrous oxide*

- **Schrader valve colour:** blue
- **Hose colour:** blue
- **Supply pressure:** 400 kPa.

Nitrous oxide is most commonly supplied from a cylinder manifold. Some theatres do not have outlets for nitrous oxide pipelines, in which case it is only available from gas cylinders on the anaesthetic machine itself.

1.2.1.4. *Piped medical vacuum*

- **Schrader valve colour:** yellow
- **Hose colour:** yellow
- **Supply pressure:** –53 kPa.

A centralized vacuum pump creates a negative pressure within the pipeline supply that is most commonly used to drive suction devices in theatre.

1.2.2 **Gas cylinders**

Gas cylinders are used to supply gases where there is no piped medical gas supply. There should also always be an oxygen cylinder on the anaesthetic machine, to be used in the event of an oxygen pipeline supply failure. Examples are pictured in Figs 1.2a and 1.2b.

Gas cylinders are made of a steel alloy, colour-coded, and clearly labelled with their contents. The valve block on top of the cylinder, where it connects to the anaesthetic machine, has a series of notches cut into it. These match pegs on the mounting on the back of the anaesthetic machine. This is termed the 'pin-index system', and each gas has a unique pin layout. This minimizes the risk of a cylinder being misconnected to the anaesthetic machine. There also needs to be a Bodok seal, a rubber ring-like device that sits between the cylinder and the inlet of the machine, ensuring a good seal.

Medical gas cylinders come in a variety of sizes. The cylinders on the anaesthetic machine are usually size E, which have an internal volume of around 4.7 L. The gases within are pressurized to a varying degree. Some details about medical gas cylinders are listed as follows:

- **Oxygen:** cylinder colour—black body with a white neck; contains only gaseous oxygen and is pressurized to 13 700 kPa when full

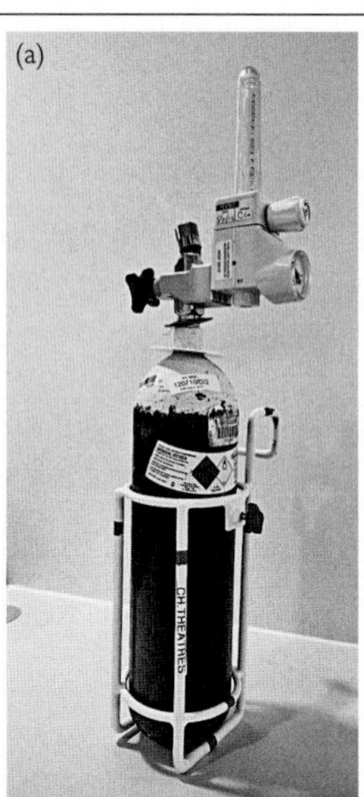

Fig 1.2a This illustrates a traditional-style cylinder. The valve assembly at the top, where the flowmeter is located, is detachable and has a pin-index system to ensure correct connection. The cylinder has a black body and white shoulders, indicating its contents to be oxygen. The plastic disc visible at the cylinder neck contains details of when the cylinder was last tested. The cylinder is manufactured from molybdenum steel and is comparatively heavy.

- **Medical air:** cylinder colour—grey body with black and white shoulders; contains only gaseous air and is pressurized to 13 700 kPa when full
- **Nitrous oxide:** cylinder colour—blue with blue neck; contains both liquid and gaseous nitrous oxide and is pressurized to around 4400 kPa.

Cylinders that contain only gases (oxygen and medical air) obey Boyle's Law, which states that the pressure of a gas multiplied by its volume is a constant. As cylinder contents are drawn off, the pressure in the cylinder falls linearly, e.g. if the pressure in an oxygen cylinder reads 13 700 kPa, it is full. If later it reads 6850 kPa, then half of its contents have been used. A full size E oxygen cylinder should deliver around 640 L of gas.

Nitrous oxide is a little different to this, since it contains both liquid and gaseous nitrous oxide. As the cylinder is used, the gaseous nitrous oxide is drawn off, which causes some of the liquid to evaporate to replace it. This means that the pressure in a nitrous oxide cylinder remains relatively constant until all the liquid has been evaporated. This only occurs when the cylinder is nearly empty. The practical consequence of this is that you cannot tell how much remains in a nitrous oxide cylinder by reading its pressure gauge, but instead the cylinder must be weighed to estimate the liquid volume remaining.

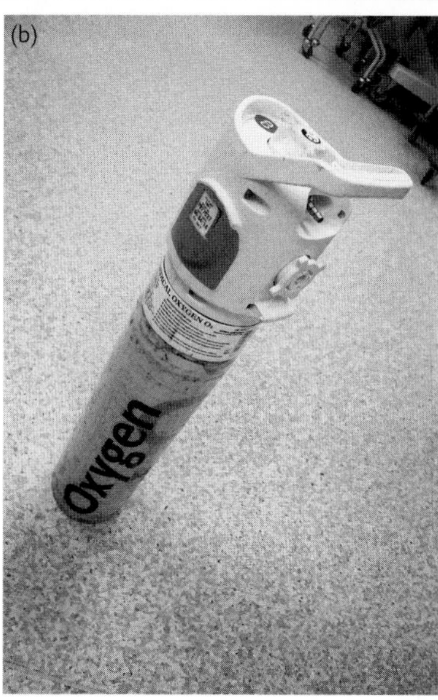

Fig 1.2b Lightweight cylinders are coloured differently to traditional devices but are still clearly marked with their contents. They are manufactured from an aluminium alloy, with a fibreglass jacket to improve portability, while the flat base makes it easier to stand them on a surface. A valve on the side of the cylinder turns the system on or off, and two different connections are visible in this image. The topmost connection, just beneath the carry handle, is suitable for connection to a face mask, using standard tubing. Gas flow to this is selected using the dial on the very top of the cylinder. The round socket below the tubing connection is a Schrader valve, into which a portable ventilator may be connected.

1.2.3 **Pressure gauges**

Pressure gauges are found on the front of the anaesthetic machine. Older machines have Bourdon gauges. These are analogue dials that denote pressure, while newer machines display pressures electronically.

The value displayed is a gauge pressure (rather than absolute pressure). Various units of pressure are used in different areas of anaesthetic practice, although the SI unit of pressure is the pascal. Some of these units are described in Table 1.1.

Gauges must be present that show pipeline pressures for each gas and also for each cylinder present. This means that the anaesthetist can ensure that sufficient gases are being delivered to the anaesthetic machine.

1.2.4 **Pressure regulators**

Pressure regulators are present in the anaesthetic machine to reduce the pressure of gases before they are delivered to the patient. Gases taken from the hospital pipeline are typically around 400 kPa; the pressure that can be safely applied to a patient's lungs should not exceed around 3 kPa.

Table 1.1 Units of pressure measurement			
Unit	Abbreviation	Atmospheric pressure (approximate)	Notes
Atmosphere	atm	1 atm	This unit is seldom used in anaesthetic practice and is not an SI unit.
Bar	bar	1 bar	Although not an SI unit, bar is commonly used when describing higher pressure gas supplies such as piped medical gases.
Kilopascal	kPa	101 kPa	The SI unit of pressure is the pascal (Pa). This is a small unit, so pressures are more commonly expressed as kPa (x 10^3 Pa). The kPa is frequently used when describing higher pressure gas supplies.
Centimetres of water	cmH_2O	1020 cmH_2O	This unit is commonly used to describe low-pressure systems, including airway pressures, and some physiological measurements such as intracranial pressure (ICP).
Millimetres of mercury	mmHg	762 mmHg	This unit is most frequently encountered in the measurement of arterial or venous blood pressures.

Pressures measured in the breathing circuit, to which the patient is attached, are generally measured in centimetres of water (cmH_2O), since the pressures that are used are much lower than those encountered in the pipelines. Atmospheric pressure is approximately 1020 cmH_2O, so 1 kPa = 10.2 cmH_2O.

1.2.5 **The flowmeter**

The flowmeter, sometimes also called a Rotameter®—the brand name of one particular device—is a means of controlling the flow of gas delivered to the breathing circuit. It can be either physical or electronic.

A physical flowmeter, illustrated in Fig 1.3, consists of a glass tube with a bobbin inside it, controlled by a knob. The diameter and shape of the tube are gas-specific; movement of the bobbin is dependent on the physical properties of the gas, particularly its viscosity and density. The meter is labelled and colour-coded, as are the control knobs.

On British anaesthetic machines, oxygen is traditionally the left-most knob and the control is often larger and of different shape. The oxygen can therefore be located by touch, should theatre lights fail. This is not always the case on machines designed in other countries.

As the knob is turned gas flows up the tube from bottom to top; this floats the bobbin within the gas stream. The bobbin moves higher as flow increases. The meter, which is calibrated in either mL/min or L/min, is read from the top of the bobbin against a scale marked on the tube.

An electronic device represents a computer-controlled valve system within the machine that is software-controlled. The machine will display the flow rate of each gas on either an LED display or an LCD screen.

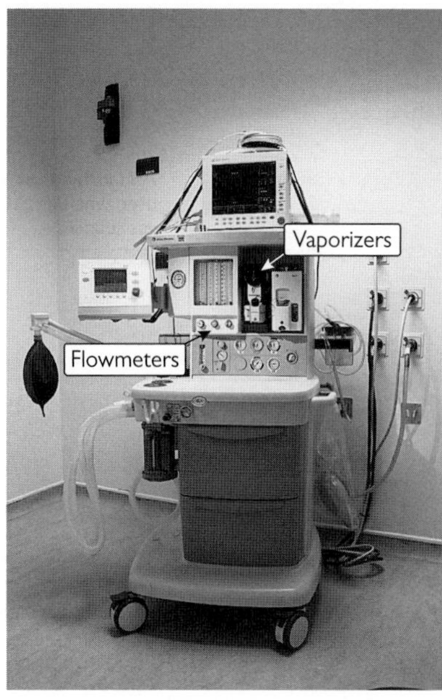

Fig 1.3 This image of an anaesthetic machine demonstrates the position of the flowmeter controls and the vaporizers.

Whichever type of flowmeter is employed there must be a system that prevents the machine from delivering a hypoxic gas mixture. This is a mixture that contains <21% oxygen (the concentration of oxygen found in atmospheric air).

1.2.6 **Anaesthetic vaporizers**

Inhalational anaesthetics, agents such as isoflurane or sevoflurane, are supplied as liquids that must be converted into the gaseous state (vaporized) to be administered to the patient. Vaporizers are the devices that are designed to achieve this.

Although the vaporizer is agent-specific, they all share common features. They must contain a tank (the vaporization chamber) to hold the liquid agent and a system for exposing that liquid to the gas flow from the flowmeters. There is also a dial that can be set by the anaesthetist to select how much agent is added to the gas flow. This is calibrated in the percentage of the volume of gas. Most anaesthetic machines can mount more than one vaporizer at a time—Fig 1.3 shows a sevoflurane and an isoflurane vaporizer mounted side by side—but there should be a system that prevents more than one vaporizer being switched on simultaneously. Vaporizers are colour-coded to show which gas they contain. Isoflurane vaporizers are marked in purple, sevoflurane in yellow, and desflurane in blue. These are illustrated in Figs 1.4a–c.

The vaporizer also has a large copper jacket that acts as a heat sink. It requires energy, in the form of latent heat of evaporation, to convert a liquid anaesthetic to the gaseous

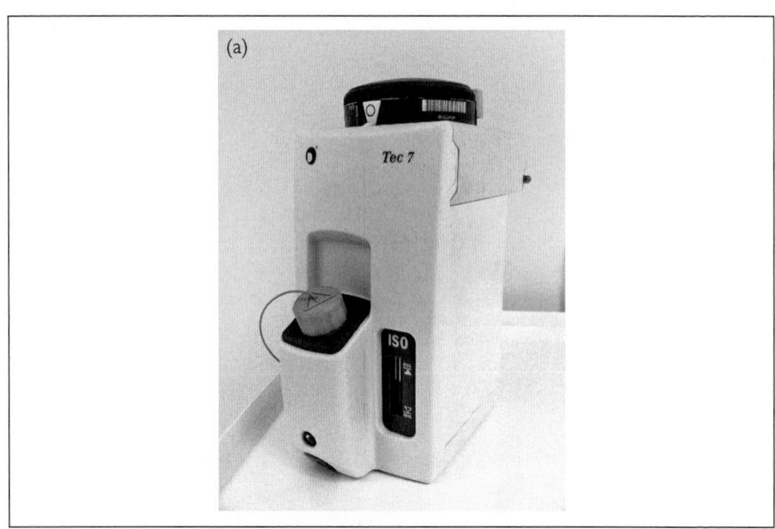

Fig 1.4a This is a Tec7 isoflurane vaporizer, manufactured by GE. The contents are identifiable by the purple colour coding, while the gauge on the right side of the filling cap indicates how full the device is.

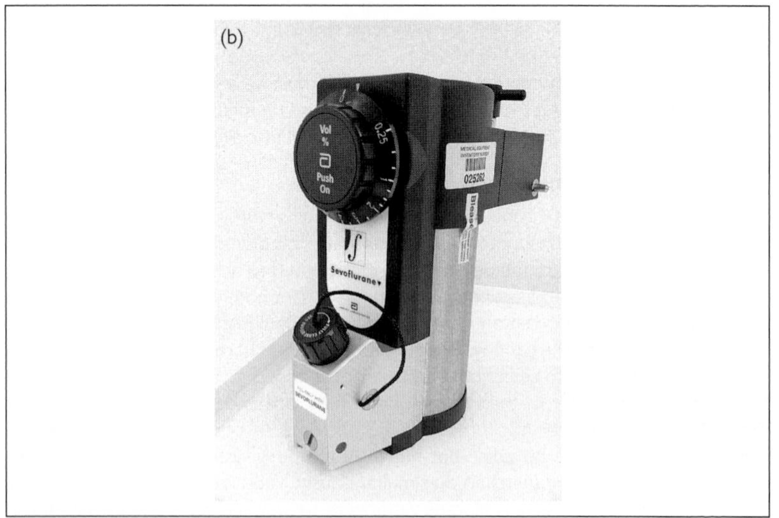

Fig 1.4b Yellow-coded vaporizers contain sevoflurane. The contents gauge is just out of sight on the left underneath the filling cap.

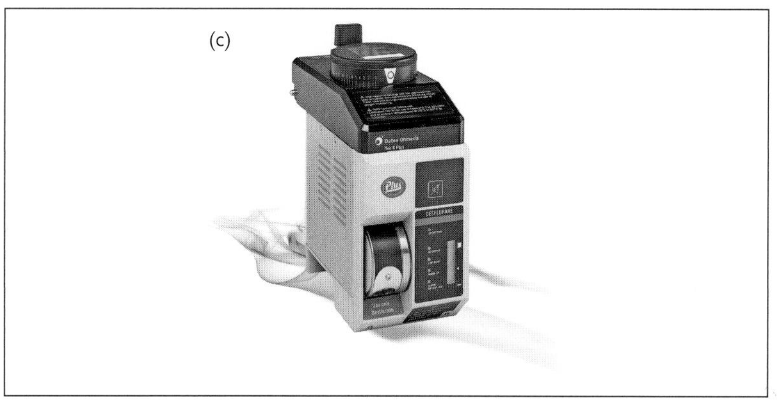

Fig 1.4c A Tec 6 Plus vaporizer. The desflurane vaporizer, colour-coded blue, differs from standard designs because of the unusual physical properties of desflurane. Unlike other agents, desflurane must be heated, so the vaporizer requires mains power.

Reproduced with kind permission of GE Medical Systems Ltd.

state. In the absence of a heat sink, the contents of the vaporizer would cool down as this latent heat is 'used up'. This would reduce the amount of anaesthetic agent evaporating, thus making the vaporizer performance unpredictable. By including a heat sink, there is effectively a reserve of heat energy available that can reduce temperature fluctuations within the system.

The gas from the flowmeters, or fresh gas flow (FGF), is divided into two streams when it enters the vaporizer. One stream bypasses the vaporization chamber completely so remains free of agent. The other stream passes through the chamber and leaves it fully saturated with agent. The amount by which this stream is diluted by the gas from the bypass channel determines the percentage of agent delivered to the patient.

1.2.6.1 *Desflurane*

The inhalational agent desflurane is handled a little differently. Desflurane has unique properties that require a vaporizer of different design. Since the boiling point of desflurane is close to room temperature (22.8°C), if it were placed in a traditional vaporizer, its output would vary greatly with small changes in temperature, making the vaporizer's performance unpredictable. To compensate for this, a desflurane vaporizer contains a computerized control system and a heating element that raises the temperature of the liquid agent to a constant 39°C, boiling the liquid inside. This produces a stream of pure desflurane gas that can be added to the FGF by computer-controlled valves. Since the desflurane is boiled in this way, this vaporizer does not need to split the incoming FGF in the manner of more traditional vaporizers.

Although the operation of the desflurane vaporizer is essentially the same as more traditional types, some models must be plugged into a power supply. When first switched on, these require a short period of time to warm up to operating temperature.

1.2.7 The common gas outlet

The common gas outlet (CGO) is the port, found usually on the front of the anaesthetic machine, to which the breathing circuit is connected. By the time the gas flow has reached this point, all the different components (oxygen, air, or nitrous oxide, and inhalational agent) have been added and mixed. The pressure of the gas flow has also been reduced to the point it can safely be delivered to the patient.

Some anaesthetic machines have a second auxiliary CGO (seen in Fig 1.5) to allow the anaesthetist to connect a different type of breathing circuit to the machine. These allow the connection of, for example, a Mapleson F breathing system for paediatric use, in addition to a built-in circle system. Such anaesthetic machines have a switch that allows the anaesthetist to select which CGO the gas stream is directed to. The anaesthetist must be in no doubt which CGO the gas is being sent to; if the patient is connected to the wrong circuit, they will receive no oxygen and no anaesthetic.

1.2.8 High-flow oxygen flush

This is a button that sends a high flow of oxygen (around 40 L/min) to the CGO. This flush bypasses the flowmeters; the gas stream does not have air or nitrous oxide mixed into it nor does it pass through the vaporizer, so it contains no anaesthetic agent. It is generally used to refill the breathing circuit reservoir bag in the event of it deflating after a leak. If it is used incautiously, there is a risk of diluting the anaesthetic gases in the breathing circuit, with a chance that the patient may become aware. The high flows can generate pressures that could traumatize the patient's lungs.

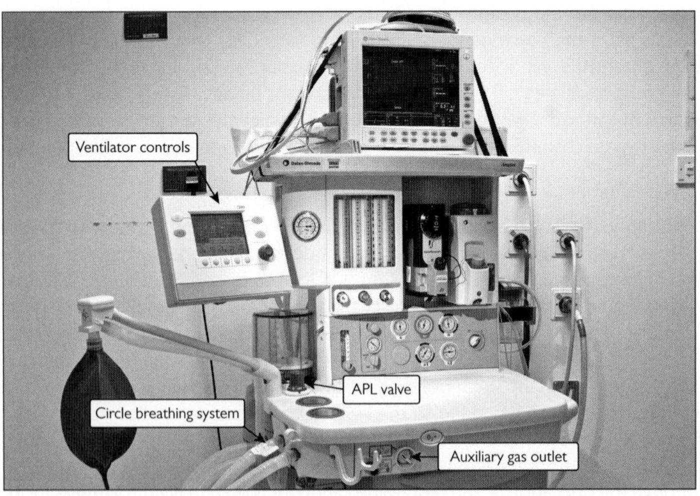

Fig 1.5 This image of a Datex Aespire anaesthetic machine shows the position of the APL valve and the breathing circuit. This type of anaesthetic machine also has an auxiliary gas outlet, the control for which is on the front of the machine near the oxygen flush button. It is important to check the switch is directing gas to the correct outlet before connecting a patient.

1.2.9 **Breathing circuits**

The term breathing circuit describes the system of hoses that carry gas from the CGO of the anaesthetic machine to the patient's airway.

There are two main classifications of breathing circuit: rebreathing systems and non-rebreathing systems. Rebreathing systems are subgrouped by the Mapleson classification, which describes six systems labelled A to F, depending on where in the circuit the fresh gas is added in relation to the expiratory valve and the patient's airway. The category of non-rebreathing systems contains only one type of circuit called a circle system.

All circuits share the same basic components: a conduit to carry gas to the airway, a reservoir bag to allow manual ventilation, and an exhaust for waste gas. In most circuits, the exhaust has an automatic pressure-limiting (APL) valve to control the pressure within the breathing circuit.

1.2.9.1 *Rebreathing systems*

With a rebreathing-type system, there must be a high flow of gas supplied from the CGO to wash out the carbon dioxide (CO_2) exhaled by the patient. If the flow is inadequate, the patient may rebreathe their expired CO_2, which may have adverse effects on their biochemistry. How much gas must be supplied varies, depending on the circuit type and whether the patient is self-ventilating or if the anaesthetist is ventilating them.

The most commonly encountered rebreathing systems are the Mapleson D (Bain circuit), often found on the anaesthetic machine in the anaesthetic room, and the Mapleson C (Waters bag). The Mapleson C is often used as an alternative means to ventilate a patient for transfer or as a backup circuit in the event of machine failure. The Mapleson F circuit is particularly used in paediatric practice, as it presents low resistance to respiration and has a particularly low circuit dead space. These circuits are illustrated in Figs 1.6a–c.

The Mapleson D system needs an FGF of 2–4 times the patient's minute volume (10 L/min or more in an average-sized adult) to prevent rebreathing. Appropriate flows for a Mapleson C system would be 1.5–2 times the minute volume (see Box 1.1).

1.2.9.2 *Circle systems*

The main feature of the circle system is that there is a canister that contains soda lime, a mixture of sodium and calcium hydroxide. This reacts with the patient's exhaled CO_2,

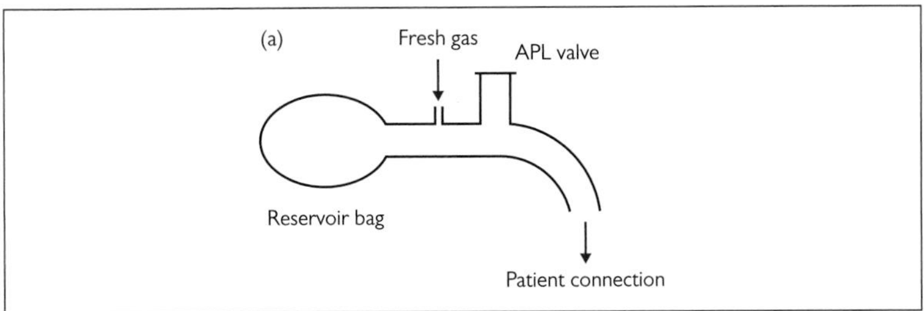

Fig 1.6a The Mapleson C system (Waters bag) is a compact and portable system useful for patient transfer, but the lack of a self-inflating bag limits its use in resuscitation.

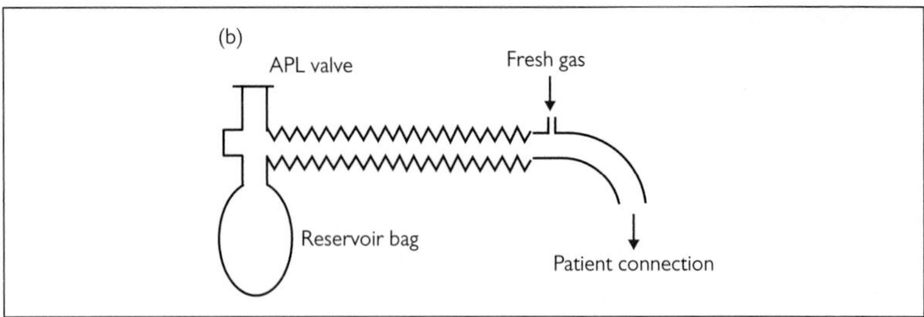

Fig 1.6b A Mapleson D system (also called a Bain circuit) is commonly used in the anaesthetic room, as it is mechanically simple and moderately efficient during manual ventilation.

removing it from the gas stream. Inhalational anaesthetics are minimally metabolized and so are present unchanged in exhaled gas, along with any excess oxygen that the patient did not need for metabolism. By removing CO_2 from the exhaled volume, the oxygen and anaesthetic can be recycled and sent back to the patient. This enables the anaesthetist to use lower FGFs, making savings in gas and agent consumption. To use a circle system safely, there must be monitoring of the gas composition at the patient's airway. In theory, it is possible to use flows as low as 250 mL/min, although it is more usual to use flow rates of around 1 L/min.

1.2.10 **The ventilator**

The ventilator is provided to allow for prolonged mechanical ventilation of the anaesthetized patient. A variety of different types of ventilator are available; they can be mechanical, pneumatic, or electronically controlled.

Most ventilators can be set to 'volume control' or 'pressure control', which determines how each breath is delivered. The system will also have a control that determines respiratory frequency.

More sophisticated ventilators also allow the anaesthetist to finely control inspiratory and expiratory times (I:E ratio) and the waveform of each delivered breath. An I:E ratio of between 1:1.5 and 1:2 is usually appropriate. Other settings rarely need to be adjusted in routine use.

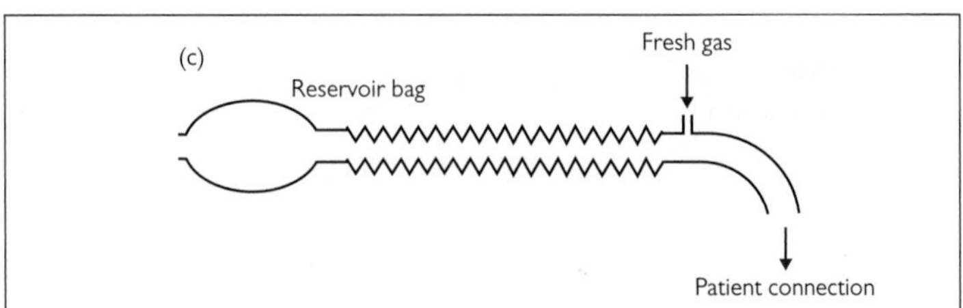

Fig 1.6c This Mapleson F system is reserved for use in small children (<20 kg). It has no valves, which means resistance, and therefore work of breathing, is very low.

Box 1.1 Definition of minute volume

Minute volume (MV) is given by **tidal volume** (V_t) multiplied by respiratory **frequency** (f).

$MV = V_t \times f$

1.2.10.1 *Volume control*

In this mode, the anaesthetist sets the tidal volume and frequency that are desired; the machine will deliver the set volume, using whatever pressure is required (subject to safety limits set by the machine). In this mode, the minute volume is constant, as it is fixed by the rate and volume chosen. There is the risk that, if the patient's respiratory compliance changes over the course of the operation (e.g. by changes in position or pneumoperitoneum at laparoscopy), the airway pressures can vary greatly.

For an average-sized adult, a tidal volume of 500 mL and a respiratory rate of 12 breaths/min, giving a minute volume of 6 L/min, are usually appropriate. These settings would usually require airway pressures of 20–30 cmH_2O. Prolonged exposure to airway pressures above 30 cmH_2O can increase the risk of pneumothorax or barotrauma to the patient's lungs. Spikes in airway pressures are also hazardous.

1.2.10.2 *Pressure control*

In this mode, the anaesthetist sets the desired inspiratory pressure and frequency. The volume delivered depends on the respiratory compliance, and therefore tidal volume (and thus minute volume) can vary over the duration of the case, depending on neuromuscular blockade, patient position, and surgical factors.

The advantage of pressure control is that, except under unusual circumstances, the airway pressures should never exceed selected limits, protecting the patient against barotrauma. This is the preferred method of ventilating paediatric cases.

1.3 Airway management

Anaesthetic agents generally depress respiration and reduce muscle tone in the airway. Much of the anaesthetist's skill rests on managing the consequences of this, and there is a range of devices available to use.

Breathing circuits all terminate in standard 22 mm connector for adult use and have an internal diameter of 15 mm suitable for connection to paediatric devices. These connectors allow for the fitting of either face masks or connection to devices such as the laryngeal mask or tracheal tube.

1.3.1 Face masks

Face masks are one of the simplest and least invasive airway devices. Usually made of plastic, they have a soft cuff around the edge to help maintain an airtight seal (see Fig 1.7). They come in a range of sizes to fit children and adults.

A well-fitting face mask should form a good seal around the mouth and nose, without excessive pressure on the patient's soft tissues. It should not make contact with the eyes.

1.3.2 Oropharyngeal airway

This is commonly referred to as a Guedel® airway, after a popular brand of the device. Examples can be seen in Fig 1.8.

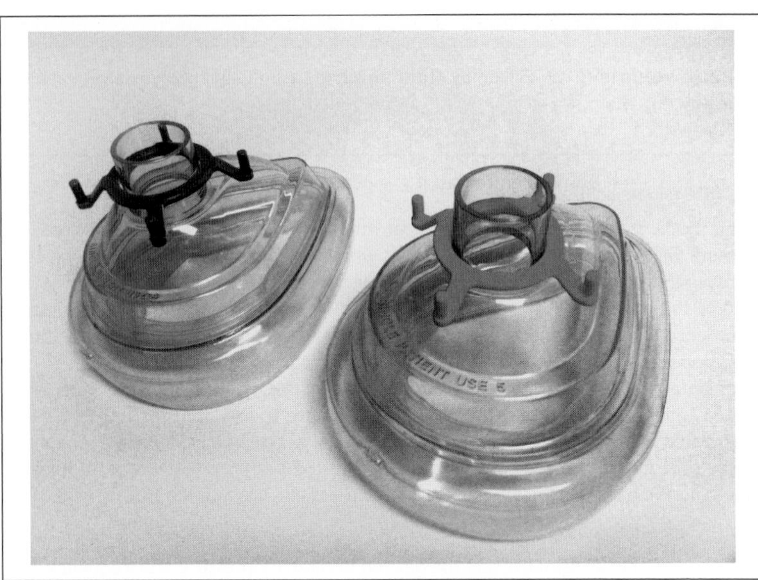

Fig 1.7 Standard face masks. The soft cuff ensures a good seal whilst minimizing pressure on the patient's face. The coloured rings denote the size of the mask. Although very rarely used, the plastic rings can be used with a specially designed harness to hold the mask to the patient's face.

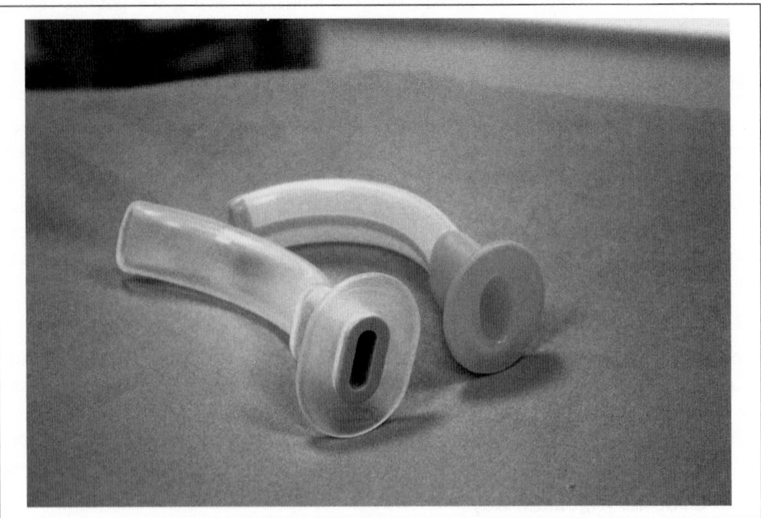

Fig 1.8 Oropharyngeal airways. Colour coding denotes the size of the airway.

Again a range of sizes is available, but generally sizes 3 to 5 are suitable for adults. They are placed in the mouth to help lift the tongue away from the posterior pharyngeal wall.

They are sized from the angle of the jaw, such that the flat portion of the airway rests between the patient's incisors, and are first inserted upside down before being rotated into position.

The presence of an airway is profoundly stimulating, and the patient must be anaesthetized before they will tolerate this. If the patient begins to cough or retch, it should be removed.

1.3.3 **Laryngeal mask airway**

The laryngeal mask airway, or LMA, is a commonly encountered device in anaesthetic practice. It possesses advantages over the simple face mask, and it is both easier to insert and less traumatic for the patient than a tracheal tube.

The LMA performs essentially the same task as a simple face mask, forming a soft seal around the patient's larynx, but, because it sits in the patient's mouth, it does not require the anaesthetist to constantly hold it, freeing them up for other tasks.

Several manufacturers produce LMAs, and they differ slightly in their form, but all share the same basic features: a standard connector at one end and at the other a soft cuff that must be inflated to form a seal (see Fig 1.9).

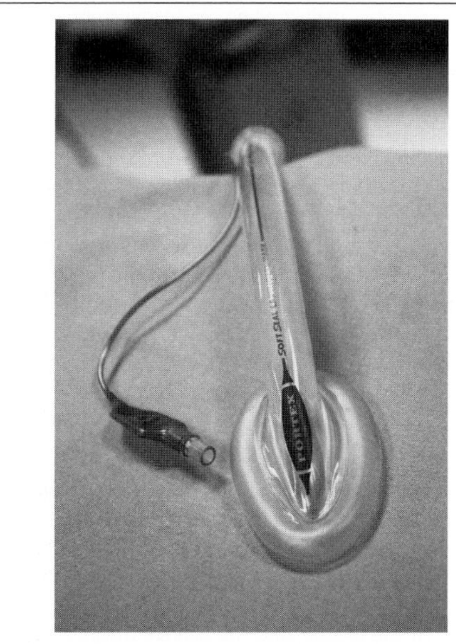

Fig 1.9 A laryngeal mask airway. The orange connector to the left of the image is used to inflate the cuff. The blue pilot balloon, just proximal to the connector, inflates with the cuff to indicate when it has been filled. The blue line along the length of the airway should line up with the patient's nose after insertion so it can be used to indicate if the airway has been displaced.

A variety of sizes are available that are suitable for children or adults. Generally, size 4 is used for women and size 5 for men. They are sized according to the patient's weight, and each size requires a different volume to fully inflate the cuff.

Although they are much less traumatic than tracheal intubation, LMAs are not suitable for every patient. Since the cuff forms an imperfect seal at the larynx, they are less suitable for patients in whom higher pressures are required to inflate the lungs. This might include obese or pregnant patients, or those with pathological conditions such as acute severe asthma or anaphylaxis. Similarly, the imperfect seal cannot fully protect the patient's airway from soiling by gastric contents, so they would not be routinely used in patients in whom there is a risk of aspiration.

1.3.4 **Tracheal tubes**

The tracheal tube is a means of providing a secure airway that protects the patient's respiratory system from foreign bodies such as gastric contents or blood. A tracheal tube provides a tight seal that facilitates mechanical ventilation with higher pressures than can be delivered with an LMA. Additionally, when affixed to the patient appropriately, it is less likely to displace or obstruct than an LMA.

There are certain disadvantages to using a tracheal tube. It takes considerably more skill to successfully place than an LMA, and intubation can potentially cause dental, oral, or laryngeal trauma. A number of deaths have been reported from unrecognized misplacement of a tracheal tube, mainly when it is inadvertently placed in the patient's oesophagus. For this reason, it is important to confirm the position of the tube after every intubation by observing chest movement, listening for bilateral breath sounds, and by measuring end-tidal CO_2.

Tracheal tubes (see Fig 1.10) come in a range of different shapes, suitable for oral or nasal insertion, and they can be reinforced with a metal wire to prevent kinking. Most tracheal tubes for adult use have a cuff to provide a seal (which requires much smaller volumes to inflate than an LMA cuff) and a standard circuit connector. Tracheal tubes come in sizes 2.5 to 9. The size refers to the internal diameter in millimetres. A size 9 tube has an internal diameter of 9 mm. Sizes 7–8 would be suitable for oral intubation of an average-sized adult woman, and sizes 8–9 would be suitable for an average adult male. Sizes 6–7 are generally suitable for nasal use in adults.

1.3.5 **Laryngoscopes**

The laryngoscope is a device used to manipulate the patient's airway to enable the anaesthetist to view the laryngeal inlet. It consists of a handle (which usually contains a battery and a light source) and a blade that is inserted into the airway.

The most commonly encountered laryngoscope blade in adult practice is the MacIntosh, usually of size 3 or 4 (see Fig 1.11a). This is inserted into the right-hand side of the patient's mouth and advanced until the tip of the epiglottis is seen. The tongue is then swept to the left of the mouth, and the handle of the laryngoscope lifted up to view the larynx.

Alternative laryngoscopes are sometimes used in the management of patients with difficult airways (see Section 7.2). Examples include the McCoy and the Polio. The McCoy blade (see Fig 1.11b) has a hinged tip that can be lifted up further by depressing

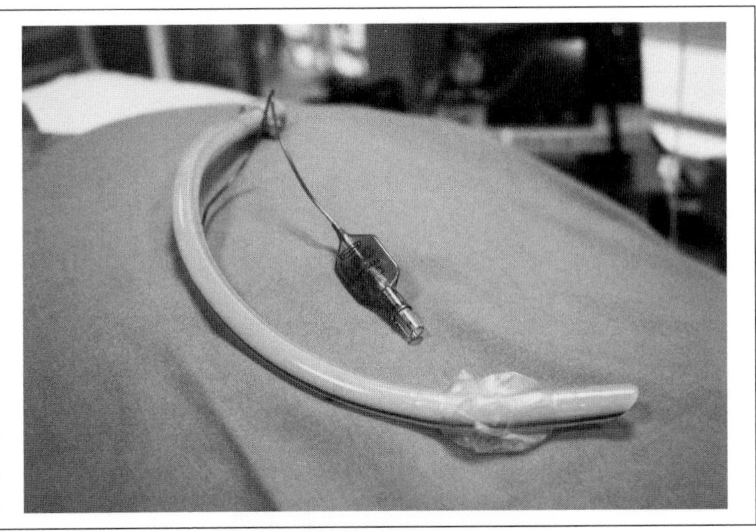

Fig 1.10 A standard tracheal tube. As with the LMA, the connector and pilot balloon allow inflation of the cuff. When placed in the trachea, the inflated cuff will form a watertight and gas-tight seal, securing the airway against aspiration.

a lever on the handle. This can be a useful device where the laryngoscopy view is poor. A Polio blade is a standard blade mounted at a steeper angle on the handle. This has value where access to the patient's mouth may be restricted, e.g. in the obese patient or pregnant woman where breast tissue may make it difficult to insert a standard blade into the mouth.

A number of video-assisted laryngoscopes are available. These have either a small video camera at the tip or a series of reflectors to enable the anaesthetist to see the larynx indirectly.

Straight-bladed laryngoscopes, such as the Magill, are occasionally used in paediatric practice. The epiglottis in children has a different shape, and the straight blade is designed to account for this.

1.3.6 **Laryngoscopy grade**

The view seen at laryngoscopy is described by the Cormack–Lehane laryngoscopy grade, which is scored depending on the amount of the larynx that can be visualized (see Fig 1.12). It is important when recording this grade that the equipment used is noted, especially if a non-standard laryngoscope or technique were used.

- **Grade I:** all of the laryngeal structures can be seen
- **Grade II:** only the posterior third of the vocal cords and the arytenoids can be seen
- **Grade III:** only the epiglottis can be seen
- **Grade IV:** no laryngeal structures can be seen.

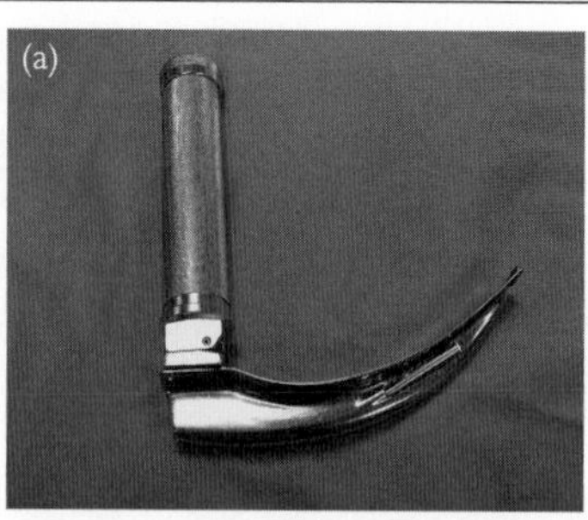

Fig 1.11a A MacIntosh laryngoscope. This is the most commonly used device for direct laryngoscopy in adults. It consists of batteries held in the handle and a light source that projects over the length of the blade.

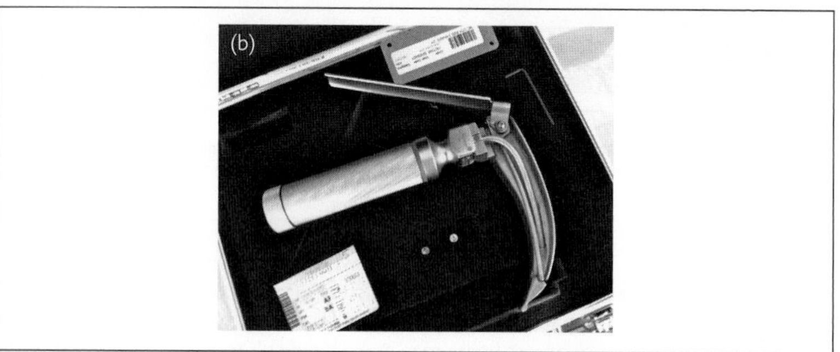

Fig 1.11b A McCoy laryngoscope in its transport case. The blade is the same shape as a MacIntosh, but the handle at the top of the image can be depressed, causing the tip of the blade to hinge upwards. This can improve the laryngoscopy view in difficult intubations.

Grade III or IV views at laryngoscopy would be termed difficult. If it is not possible to place the tracheal tube successfully, it may be necessary to follow a failed intubation drill (see Section 7.2).

1.4 Monitoring equipment

It is important that the patient is appropriately monitored whilst undergoing anaesthesia. A specific 'minimum monitoring standard' is nationally recognized. If an item of monitoring is not available, it may be appropriate to continue with the case, but a senior anaesthetist should make this decision and the reason documented in the case notes.

The Association of Anaesthetists of Great Britain and Ireland (AAGBI) have set the minimum monitoring standard for general anaesthesia in a fit adult patient as:

- Oxygen saturation
- Electrocardiography

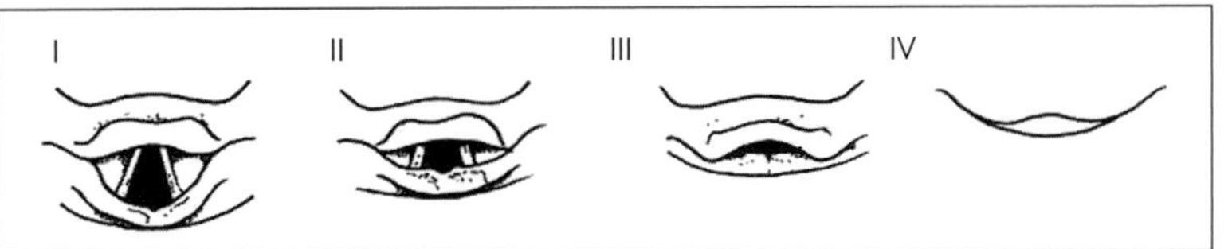

Fig 1.12 Cormack and Lehane grading for the structures seen at direct laryngoscopy.
Reproduced from Allman and Wilson, *Oxford Handbook of Anaesthesia* 3rd edition, 2011, page 971 with permission from Oxford University Press.

- Non-invasive blood pressure (NIBP)
- End-tidal capnography
- Anaesthetic agent monitoring
- Airway pressure.

Other items of equipment must be immediately available but may not be necessary in all cases. These might include temperature monitoring and a peripheral nerve stimulator (mandatory for any patient that has received a muscle relaxant).

1.4.1 **Oxygen saturation**

Oxygen saturation is measured by pulse oximetry. The pulse oximeter is an electronic device that calculates the percentage of oxygenated haemoglobin present in arterial blood. The system is based on the differential absorption of red light at two different wavelengths (660 nm and 940 nm) by oxyhaemoglobin and deoxyhaemoglobin. The signal processor in the oximeter measures the total absorption of the light in all the tissue and then subtracts the non-pulsatile component from the measurement; this excludes the light absorbed by venous blood and by tissues, leaving only the arterial component.

There are potential sources of error in this measurement; chiefly its accuracy is dependent on good tissue perfusion; thus, if blood supply to the part of the body where the probe is located is poor, the device is likely to give an erroneous reading. High ambient light can swamp the detectors and movement can be mistakenly read as pulsatile signal, which can also yield errors.

Most anaesthetic monitors also include a visual representation of the pulsatile signal the machine is reading. If this trace is of a poor quality, the reading is more likely to be inaccurate.

1.4.2 **Electrocardiography**

Continuous three-lead electrocardiogram (ECG) monitoring is required during all anaesthetic cases. The ECG records electrical impulses that originate in the heart by measuring potential differences between different parts of the body. These potential differences are around 1 mV at the skin.

Electrodes are placed on each shoulder and one on the left mid-axillary line. This lead placement allows the recording of leads I, II, and III; typically, lead II is displayed on the monitor, as the P waves are upright and the QRS complexes are isoelectric.

ECG monitor errors can arise from patient movement, since the electrical potentials generated by muscles are of much greater magnitude than those arising from the heart.

Interference can also come from any electrical equipment around the patient or from diathermy. If an abnormal ECG rhythm is displayed on screen, a useful check can be to look at the pulse oximeter trace—if this is still of normal character and rate, it is unlikely that there is a significant arrhythmia.

1.4.3 **Non-invasive blood pressure**

Devices to automatically measure NIBP are widely available. These devices all function by broadly similar principles, although the detail may vary from machine to machine.

NIBP monitors have an air pump to inflate the cuff above systolic blood pressure, either at the anaesthetist's command or after a specified time interval. This cuff is then slowly deflated while a pressure sensor records fluctuations in pressure transmitted from the patient's artery, analogous to Korotkoff sounds. The pressure sensor may be placed in the inflation cuff or there may be a second 'sensing cuff' incorporated into the design.

False readings of blood pressure can occur in the presence of arrhythmias, particularly atrial fibrillation (AF), since the inconsistent pulse interval leads to errors. Similarly, movement of the arm during the reading can prevent a measurement, and, if the pressure is very low, the machine may not read at all.

1.4.4 **End-tidal capnography**

Capnography is the measurement of CO_2 concentration; when measured at the end of an exhaled breath (end-tidal), the levels correlate with the patient's arterial pCO_2. Technically capnography refers to the display of this measurement as a waveform, and capnometry refers to the display of numerical value representing peak CO_2. Numerical values are displayed as a percentage. Most anaesthetic monitors display both a waveform and a value.

Two main types of capnograph device exist. These are termed mainstream analysers or side-stream analysers.

Mainstream devices require that a special piece of tubing containing a sensor be placed in the anaesthetic circuit. CO_2 absorbs infrared light, which is beamed through the breathing circuit gases by the sensor. This measurement is direct and does not require the removal of any gas from the FGF so is very quick, but the sensor can be bulky. It must be placed as close to the patient's airway as possible to provide an accurate measurement, so the additional weight does increase the risk of accidental circuit disconnection. Since water also absorbs infrared, if the sensor windows become wet, inaccurate readings may be provided. This can be an issue because the patient's exhaled breath is humid, so a filter should be placed between the sensor and the patient's airway. Mainstream analysers can only measure CO_2.

Side-stream analysers measure gas samples drawn from the breathing circuit, usually at a rate of 150 mL/min. They have the advantage that they do not require bulky equipment to be placed close to the patient's airway, and it is convenient to incorporate the system into a device to simultaneously measure anaesthetic agent concentration. The main disadvantage is a slower response time since time is taken to physically conduct the gas from the breathing circuit to the measuring device. There can be a delay of several seconds before changes are reflected on-screen. Also, not all monitors return the sampled gas to the breathing circuit, which may be an issue if the FGF is very low.

Capnography is one of the most valuable pieces of monitoring equipment. Most obviously it yields information on the adequacy of the patient's respiratory effort; CO_2 concentration is inversely proportional to the patient's minute volume, so a high CO_2 usually implies that ventilation is inadequate and vice versa.

The shape of the capnograph waveform also changes under certain pathological conditions (see Figs 1.13a–c). A slurred upstroke to the wave suggests uneven emptying of alveolar units which might imply bronchoconstriction. A sudden fall in end-tidal CO_2 is seen when blood flow to the lungs is impaired, e.g. with a rapid fall in cardiac output or after a pulmonary or air embolism. Rising CO_2 is usually caused by inadequate ventilation but may be seen in serious conditions such as malignant hyperpyrexia.

A complete absence of end-tidal CO_2 can be caused by several factors (see Section 7.3)—most commonly because the airway is misplaced or has become disconnected, or because the airway has become completely obstructed.

1.4.5 **Anaesthetic agent monitoring**

Anaesthetic agent monitoring is mandatory during cases involving inhaled anaesthetics but becomes particularly important when low gas flows are being used with a circle

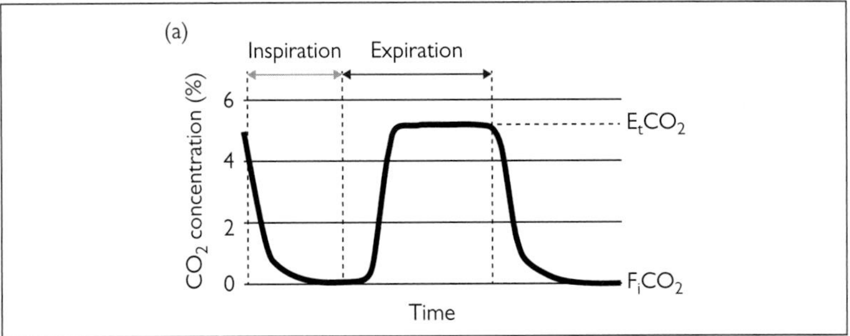

Fig 1.13a An illustration of a normal capnograph trace demonstrating inspiratory and expiratory phases of respiration. End-tidal CO_2 concentration ($EtCO_2$) can be read off the end of the expiratory plateau, while inspired CO_2 is measured at the marked point.

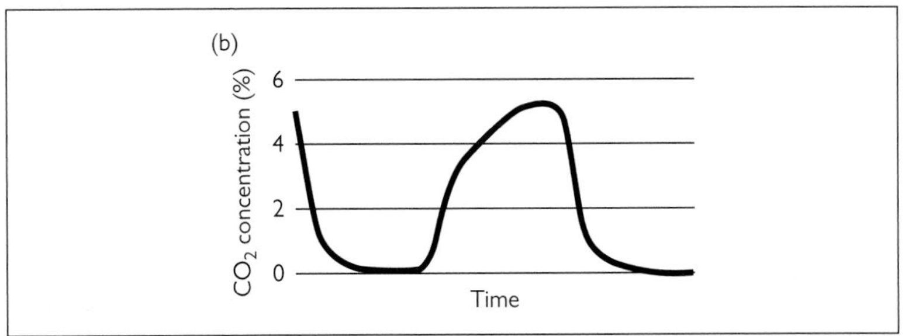

Fig 1.13b An example of a capnograph trace from a patient with bronchoconstriction. The slurred upstroke in expiration is caused by uneven emptying of alveoli supplied by narrowed bronchi.

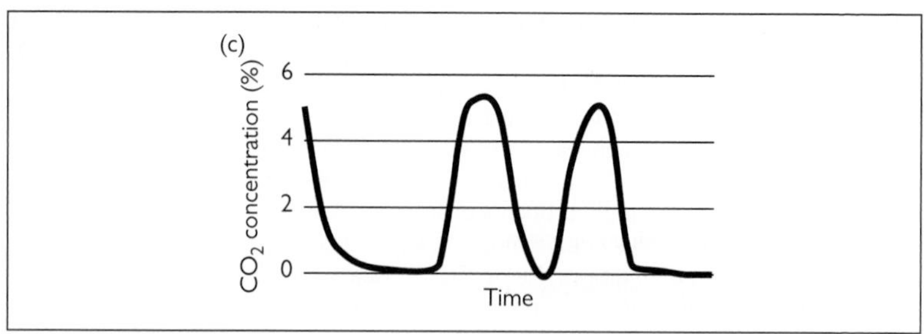

Fig 1.13c This capnograph illustrates interbreathing during mechanical ventilation. The regular pattern of inspiration and expiration has been interrupted, as the patient has taken a spontaneous breath during the ventilator expiratory phase.

breathing system. When using low flow rates on a circle system, the recycling of gases means that the concentrations of the various components delivered to the patient differ from those set on the controls of the anaesthetic machine.

Devices are usually based on either differential absorption of different light wavelengths or on mass spectroscopy.

Agent monitoring devices can be configured to display both a waveform and a numerical display of the agent's percentage concentration. Some machines will also display a minimum alveolar concentration (MAC) value. MAC values can be used as a guide to the depth of anaesthesia. MAC values have been calculated for all commonly used anaesthetic agents, although MAC values vary with patient's age and other drugs given during the anaesthetic. See Section 2.3 for more information.

1.4.6 **Airway pressure**

Airway pressures can be measured directly while flow rates are measured using a pitot tube. This device measures the drop in pressure across a specialized component in the breathing circuit. A computer can also use this information to derive tidal volume, respiratory rate, and minute volume.

Generally, the peak airway pressure should not exceed 30–40 cmH_2O to protect the patient's lungs from barotrauma. High airway pressures can be a sign of airway obstruction or bronchoconstriction (see Section 7.4).

1.5 **Machine checks**

A thorough check of anaesthetic equipment is vital before a list begins. It is the responsibility of the anaesthetist to ensure that the equipment is working correctly. Some modern anaesthetic machines include a 'self-test'. The anaesthetist is not required to repeat tests that the machine has completed, although the anaesthetist should check that the tests have been run recently.

The following sequence is taken from the AAGBI Machine Checks guidance document, reproduced in Fig 1.14 and demonstrated in Fig 1.15.

Checklist for anaesthetic equipment 2012

AAGBI safety guideline

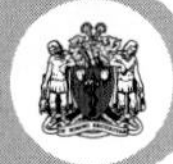

Checks at the start of every operating session
Do not use this equipment unless you have been trained

Check self-inflating bag available

Perform manufacturer's (automatic) machine check

Power supply	• Plugged in • Switched on • Backup battery charged
Gas supplies and suction	• Gas and vacuum pipelines—'tug test' • Cylinders filled and turned off • Flowmeters working (if applicable) • Hypoxic guard working • Oxygen flush working • Suction clean and working
Breathing system	• Whole system patent and leak-free using 'two-bag' test • Vaporizers—fitted correctly, filled, leak-free, plugged in (if necessary) • Soda lime—color checked • Alternative systems (Bain, T-piece)—checked • Correct gas outlet selected
Ventilator	• Working and configured correctly
Scavenging	• Working and configured correctly
Monitors	• Working and configured correctly • Alarm limits and volumes set
Airway equipment	• Full range required, working, with spares

RECORD THIS CHECK IN THE PATIENT RECORD

Don't forget!	• Self-inflating bag • Common gas outlet • Difficult airway equipment • Resuscitation equipment • TIVA and/or other infusion equipment

This guideline is not a standard of medical care. The ultimate judgement with regard to a particular clinical procedure or treatment plan must be made by the clinician in the light of the clinical data presented and the diagnostic and treatment options available.

Fig 1.14 Checklist for anaesthetic equipment (2012).

Reproduced with the kind permission of the Association of Anaesthetists of Great Britain and Ireland.

CHECKS BEFORE EACH CASE

Breathing system	Whole system patent and leak-free using 'two-bag' test Vaporizers—fitted correctly, filled, leak-free, plugged in (if necessary) Alternative systems (Bain, T-piece) – checked Correct gas outlet selected
Ventilator	Working and configured correctly
Airway equipment	Full range required, working, with spares
Suction	Clean and working

THE TWO-BAG TEST

A two-bag test should be performed after the breathing system, vaporizers, and ventilator have been checked individually

i. Attach the patient end of the breathing system (including angle piece and filter) to a test lung or bag.

ii. Set the fresh gas flow to 5 L/min and ventilate manually. Check the whole breathing system is patent and the unidirectional valves are moving. Check the function of the APL valve by squeezing both bags.

iii. Turn on the ventilator to ventilate the test lung. Turn off the fresh gas flow, or reduce to a minimum. Open and close each vaporizer in turn. There should be no loss of volume in the system.

This checklist is an abbreviated version of the publication by the Association of Anaesthetists of Great Britain and Ireland 'Checking Anaesthesia Equipment 2012'. It was originally published in *Anaesthesia*.
(Endorsed by the Chief Medical Officers)

If you wish to refer to this guideline, please use the following reference: Checklist for anaesthetic equipment 2012. *Anaesthesia* 2012; **66:** pages 662–63. <http://onlinelibrary.wiley.com/doi/10.1111/j.1365-2044.2012.07163.x/abstract>

Fig 1.14 Continued

1.5.1 **Checking an anaesthetic machine**

Before checking the machine, take note of any information or labelling on the anaesthetic machine referring to its current status. Particular attention should be paid to recent servicing. Servicing labels should be fixed in the service logbook.

1.5.1.1 *Power supply*

- Check that a mains supply is connected and turned on and that the backup batteries are charged.

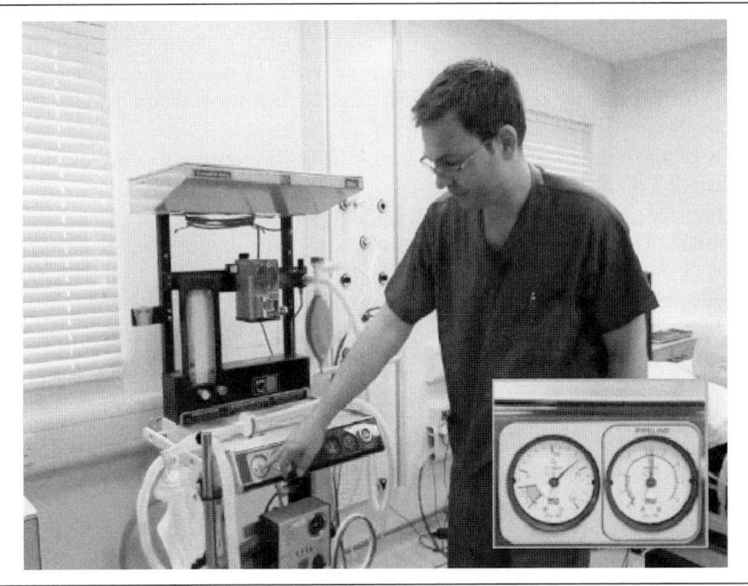

Fig 1.15 This demonstrates how to check an anaesthetic machine using the sequence taken from the Association of Anaesthetists of Great Britain and Ireland Machine Checks guidance document. There are several major steps, including power supply (00.11), gas supplies and suction (00.31), breathing system (02.39), ventilator (05.50), scavenging, monitors, and airway equipment (all at 06.44). A video of this is available in the video appendix.

1.5.1.2 *Gas supplies and suction*

- Perform a 'tug-test' on all gas and pipeline connections. Check, in particular, that the oxygen pipeline is connected and that a reserve cylinder is mounted on the machine
- Check that adequate supplies of other gases (nitrous oxide, air) are available and connected as appropriate
- Check that all pipeline pressure gauges in use on the anaesthetic machine indicate 400–500 kPa
- If flowmeters are equipped, check that each flow valve operates smoothly and that the bobbin moves freely throughout its range
- Check the anti-hypoxia device is working correctly
- Check the operation of the emergency oxygen bypass control
- Check that suction equipment is clean and operational.

1.5.1.3 *Breathing system*

Note: a new single-use bacterial/viral filter and angle-piece/catheter mount must be used for each patient. Packaging should not be removed until the point of use.

- Inspect the system for correct configuration. All connections should be secured by 'push and twist'
- Perform a pressure leak test on the breathing system by occluding the patient-end and compressing the reservoir bag. Bain-type coaxial systems should have the inner tube compressed for the leak test
- Check the correct operation of all valves, including unidirectional valves within a circle and all exhaust valves
- Check for patency and flow of gas through the whole breathing system, including the filter and angle-piece/catheter mount
- Check that each vaporizer is correctly seated on the back-bar and adequately, but not overly, filled. If a desflurane vaporizer is present, ensure it is powered
- Check each vaporizer for leaks (with vaporizer on and off) by temporarily occluding the CGO.

1.5.1.4 *Ventilator*

- Check that the ventilator tubing is correctly configured and securely attached
- Set the controls for use, and ensure that an adequate pressure is generated during the inspiratory phase
- Check the pressure relief valve functions
- Check that the disconnect alarms function correctly
- Ensure that an alternative means to ventilate the patient's lungs is available.

1.5.1.5 *Scavenging*

- Check that the tubing is attached to the appropriate exhaust port of the breathing system, ventilator, or workstation.

1.5.1.6 *Monitors*

- Check that gas sampling lines are properly attached and free of obstructions
- Check that an appropriate frequency of recording NIBP is selected
- Ensure that alarm limits are set appropriately.

1.5.1.7 *Airway equipment*

- A full range of equipment includes laryngoscopes, intubation aids, intubation forceps, bougies, face masks, airways, tracheal tubes, and connectors, in an appropriate range of sizes. Spares for each should be available.

1.5.1.8 *Other necessary equipment*

- Check that an alternative means to ventilate the patient is immediately available (e.g. self-inflating bag and oxygen cylinder)
- Check that the patient trolley, bed, or operating table can be rapidly tilted head down
- Difficult airway equipment is available
- Resuscitation equipment is available
- TIVA pumps or other infusion devices are available, as appropriate.

1.5.1.9 *Recording*

- Sign and date the logbook, kept with the anaesthetic machine, to confirm the machine has been checked
- Record on each patient's anaesthetic chart that the anaesthetic machine, breathing system, and monitoring equipment have been checked.

1.6 Self-assessment questions

Answer either true or false for each of the following questions. The answers can be found in Appendix 2.

1. **Which of the following devices are designed to minimize the risk of gas supply misconnection?**

   A. Pin-index system
   B. APL valve
   C. NIST
   D. Schrader valve
   E. Bodok seal

2. **Which of the following pressure measurements are approximations of 1 atmosphere?**

   A. 13 700 kPa
   B. 1 bar
   C. 400 kPa
   D. 762 mmHg
   E. 101 kPa

3. **Which of these airway devices would be appropriate for managing the airway of a non-fasted patient who requires an emergency anaesthetic?**

   A. Classic LMA
   B. Cuffed tracheal tube
   C. Oropharyngeal airway
   D. Hudson mask
   E. Nasal airway

4. **Concerning gas supplies in theatre:**

   A. Oxygen is carried in white hoses
   B. Air is carried in black and white hoses
   C. Nitrous oxide cylinders contain only nitrous oxide gas
   D. Nitrous oxide cylinders are blue and white
   E. Nitrous oxide is available as a piped medical gas in theatre

5. Which of the following are SI units of pressure?

   A. Pascal
   B. Bar
   C. Atmosphere
   D. Centimetre of water (cmH_2O)
   E. Millimetre of mercury (mmHg)

6. The following are types of direct laryngoscope:

   A. McCoy
   B. Polio
   C. MacIntosh
   D. Magill
   E. Davidson

7. The following are components of the Mapleson C breathing circuit:

   A. APL valve
   B. Unidirectional valves
   C. Soda lime canister
   D. 22 mm patient connector
   E. Self-inflating reservoir bag

8. Please look at Fig 1.16, and answer the following questions:

   A. The circuit illustrated would be included in the Mapleson classification
   B. The CO_2 absorber contains soda lime

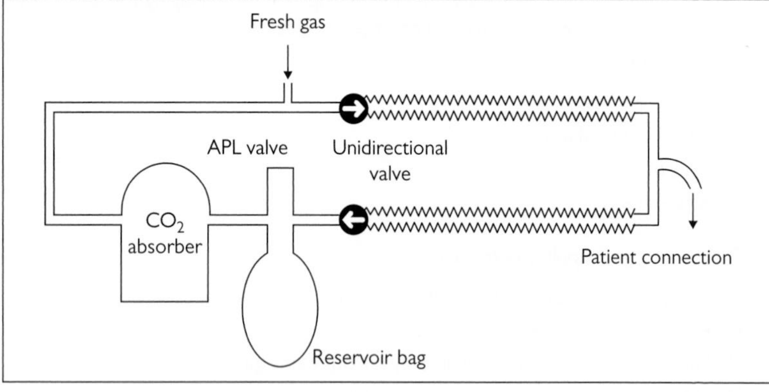

Fig 1.16 Breathing circuit.

C. This circuit would be suitable for use with small children (weighing <20 kg)

D. The circuit requires high gas flows (at least twice the patient's minute volume) to prevent rebreathing

E. Gas composition is best monitored as it leaves the CO_2 absorber

9. Which of the following are true about the Mapleson D breathing system?

A. The circuit is highly efficient in spontaneous ventilation

B. The circuit can be used at low flow rates (<1 L/min)

C. The circuit cannot be used with a mechanical ventilator

D. 2–4 times the minute volume is required in controlled ventilation to prevent rebreathing

E. A coaxial Mapleson D system is called a Bain circuit

10. Please consider the capnograph waveform in Fig 1.17:

A. A represents inspiration

B. B represents expiration

C. A rise in the value of point C is most likely to represent hypoventilation of the patient

D. A fall in the value of point D might suggest hyperventilation

E. A change in the shape of the curve at point E can be associated with pathology

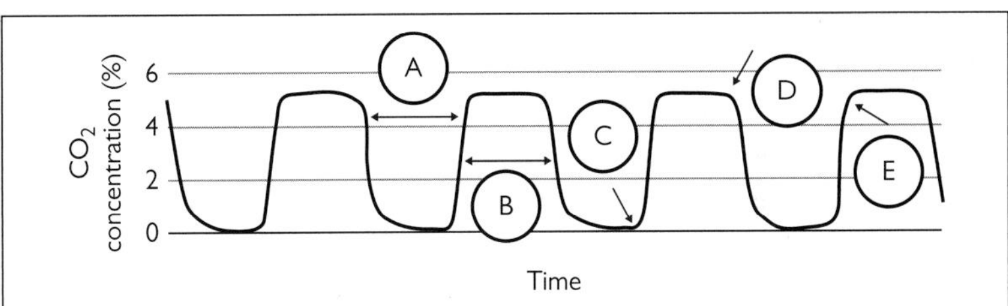

Fig 1.17 Capnograph waveform.

Chapter 2

Anaesthetic pharmacology

2.1 Introduction

Anaesthetic practice requires knowledge of a wide range of drugs, their indications, doses, and side effects. The following chapter describes some of the core drugs with which the anaesthetist must be most familiar.

2.2 Intravenous anaesthetic agents

General anaesthesia is most commonly induced using intravenous (IV) agents. Propofol has the useful property of reducing upper airway reflexes, facilitating LMA use. This is one reason that it has become the most commonly used IV anaesthetic agent.

IV agents can also be used to maintain general anaesthesia; again propofol is often the agent of choice, although sodium thiopental may be desirable under very specific circumstances.

2.2.1 Propofol

Propofol is an IV induction agent, derived from phenol. It is the most commonly used IV anaesthetic agent and can be used for induction as a single bolus or for the maintenance of anaesthesia by continuous infusion. In small doses, it can be used for conscious sedation.

Chemical name: 2,6-diisopropylphenol.

Presentation: it is highly lipid-soluble and therefore only very poorly soluble in water. It is presented as a white emulsion, with a concentration of 10 mg/mL in 20 mL ampoules. Larger 50 mL vials, with a strength of either 10 mg/mL or 20 mg/mL, are available for preparing continuous infusions.

Dose: the induction dose for propofol is 2 mg/mL.

Central nervous system (CNS): propofol causes anaesthesia within 1 arm:brain circulation time. Propofol reduces cerebral metabolism, oxygen demands, and ICP.

Respiratory: propofol is associated with reduction in respiratory drive and decreased sensitivity to CO_2.

Cardiovascular: propofol is a profound vasodilator and can also be associated with bradycardia, especially in children.

Other: propofol may have some antiemetic properties. When given by continuous infusion, may discolour urine green.

Side effects: propofol is generally a safe drug. Although allergies are very rare it does contain soya bean oil in the suspension, to which some patients are sensitive. Propofol administration, especially into small veins, can be uncomfortable or painful. Giving small amounts of lidocaine, along with the propofol dose, can reduce this.

Metabolism: patients will generally wake after around 8 min after a single 2 mg/kg dose of propofol. Although it is metabolized relatively slowly by the liver, the short duration of the clinical effect is caused by redistribution of the active drug throughout adipose tissues.

2.2.2 **Sodium thiopental**

Sodium thiopental is a potent barbiturate, which has useful properties in the induction of general anaesthesia. It is generally only used for rapid sequence induction (RSI) techniques (see Section 5.2).

Chemical name: [5-ethyl-4,6-dioxo-5-(pentan-2-yl)-1,4,5,6-tetrahydropyrimidin-2-yl]sulfanide sodium.

Presentation: supplied in glass ampoules as 500 mg of yellowish powder, for reconstitution in water or 0.9% saline.

Dose: thiopental is given in doses of 3–7 mg/kg.

CNS: thiopental will predictably induce anaesthesia in 1 arm:brain circulation time. It has a significant effect in reducing ICP and cerebral metabolism.

Respiratory: thiopental reduces respiratory drive and decreases sensitivity to CO_2.

Cardiovascular: thiopental is a myocardial depressant and vasodilator. Significant falls in blood pressure are associated with use in hypovolaemic patients, which can precipitate cardiac arrest. Care must be taken to volume-resuscitate prior to induction and to monitor blood pressure closely.

Other: thiopental does not cause pain on injection, and the dose–response is potentially more predictable than that of propofol, which may be of use when performing an RSI technique.

Side effects: allergy to thiopental is rare, but it is contraindicated in patients with porphyria. If thiopental extravasates, or if it is inadvertently injected intra-arterially, it is highly toxic and can cause significant tissue damage.

Metabolism: thiopental is seldom given by continuous infusion as its pharmacokinetics leads it to accumulate, resulting in a very slow offset time. After a single dose, patients would be expected to wake in around 8 min.

2.3 **Inhalational anaesthetic agents**

Inhalational anaesthetic agent potency is described by the concept of MAC. This reflects the amount of anaesthetic that is required to prevent an unpremedicated patient from moving to a standard surgical incision. The lower the MAC value, the more potent the agent. MAC can be used as a means of estimating the depth of anaesthesia; unless other drugs are given, the risk of awareness increases if patients are maintained with end-tidal agent concentrations below 1 MAC.

Three inhalational anaesthetics are commonly used in the United Kingdom (UK): sevoflurane, isoflurane, and desflurane. All are potential triggers of malignant hyperthermia (MH), a rare, but potentially serious, hereditary metabolic condition that is related to certain anaesthetic drugs (see Section 7.11).

2.3.1 **Sevoflurane**

Sevoflurane can be used both as an induction agent and as a means of maintaining general anaesthesia. It is somewhat more expensive than isoflurane, which limits its use in some institutions.

Chemical name: fluoromethyl-2,2,2-trifluoro-1-(trifluoromethyl) ethyl ether.

Presentation: brown glass bottles containing 250 mL of liquid agent and administered via anaesthetic vaporizer with the colour code yellow.

Dose: MAC in air of 2.00.

Respiratory: bronchodilation and dose-dependent respiratory depression.

Cardiovascular: vasodilatation and myocardial depression.

Other: sevoflurane is relatively insoluble in water and has a fast onset time. It is pleasant to breathe and is suitable for inhalational induction. More expensive than isoflurane, which sometimes limits its use in some trusts.

Side effects: potential trigger of MH.

Metabolism: only 5% is metabolized, primarily in the liver. The offset of the effect is dependent on exhalation.

2.3.2 **Isoflurane**

Isoflurane is a potent inhalational anaesthetic agent, used commonly for the maintenance of general anaesthesia. Cheaper than sevoflurane, it is widely used throughout the UK, although its pungent smell and irritant properties mean it is not suitable for inhalational induction of anaesthesia.

Chemical name: 1-chloro-2,2,2-trifluoroethyl difluoromethyl ether.

Presentation: brown glass bottles containing 250 mL of liquid agent and administered via anaesthetic vaporizer with the colour code purple.

Dose: MAC in air of 1.15.

Respiratory: bronchodilation and dose-dependent respiratory depression.

Cardiovascular: vasodilatation and myocardial depression.

Other: cheaper than sevoflurane, but can provoke coughing and laryngospasm if administered in high concentrations to lightly anaesthetized patients, so is unsuitable for inhalational inductions.

Side effects: isoflurane is a potential trigger of MH.

Metabolism: only 0.01% is metabolized, primarily in the liver. The offset of effect is dependent on exhalation.

2.3.3 Desflurane

Desflurane is an inhalational anaesthetic agent used in the maintenance of general anaesthesia. It has a pungent smell and is highly irritant in light planes of anaesthesia so is unsuitable for inhalational induction of anaesthesia. Desflurane has unusual physical properties, including a boiling point of 22.8°C, close to room temperature, requiring administration by a specialized vaporizer.

Desflurane is highly insoluble in water, which means the onset and offset time for desflurane is considerably faster than with other agents; care must be taken when adjusting desflurane vaporizer settings to achieve the desired clinical effect.

Chemical name: 2-(difluoromethoxy)-1,1,1,2-tetrafluoro-ethane.

Presentation: brown glass bottles containing 250 mL of liquid agent and administered via anaesthetic vaporizer with the colour code blue.

Dose: MAC in air of 6.35.

Respiratory: bronchodilation and dose-dependent respiratory depression. Its use is associated with breath holding, cough, and laryngospasm, especially at lighter planes of anaesthesia.

Cardiovascular: vasodilatation, myocardial depression, and tachycardia are evident at concentrations in excess of 1 MAC.

Other: desflurane is more expensive than sevoflurane and isoflurane. Its unique physical properties require a specialized vaporizer to administer. Desflurane has extremely rapid onset and offset.

Side effects: desflurane is a potential trigger of MH.

Metabolism: only 0.01% is metabolized, primarily in the liver. The offset of effect is dependent on exhalation.

2.3.4 Nitrous oxide

Nitrous oxide is a weak anaesthetic agent with a MAC of 110. Nitrous oxide is too weak an agent to achieve general anaesthesia when given as a single agent. It is commonly used as a second carrier gas, alongside oxygen, when using isoflurane or sevoflurane. When mixed with a volatile agent, their effects are additive, so a patient breathing 50% nitrous oxide will generally require only half as much volatile agent. Additionally, although nitrous oxide is a weak myocardial depressant, these effects are outweighed by slight sympathetic stimulation. The reduction in volatile agent permitted by nitrous oxide use can therefore help to provide a more cardiac-stable anaesthetic.

The chemical properties of nitrous oxide also speed the absorption of volatile agents, which can usefully shorten the duration of inhalational induction. This is termed the second gas effect. As nitrous oxide requires high concentrations to achieve useful effects it is administered by a flowmeter, rather than by a vaporizer.

Unlike other volatile agents, nitrous oxide has analgesic properties, and it also has a role to play for short-term pain relief in the emergency department, labour ward, and for dressing changes. Here, it is often presented as Entonox™, a 50:50 mixture of oxygen and nitrous oxide.

Nitrous oxide is more soluble than nitrogen in water so will tend to cause gas-filled cavities in the body to expand, as they fill with nitrous oxide faster than nitrogen can leave. Although seldom a problem in routine practice, nitrous oxide is contraindicated in patients with undrained pneumothoraces, pneumocranium, and in some ophthalmic operations.

Nitrous oxide is also associated with post-operative nausea and vomiting (PONV) and is a potent greenhouse gas.

Nitrous oxide is not a trigger agent for MH.

Chemical name: dinitrogen monoxide.

2.4 Muscle relaxants and reversal agents

2.4.1 Non-depolarizing neuromuscular blockade

Non-depolarizing neuromuscular-blocking drugs act by competitive inhibition of acetylcholine at nicotinic acetylcholine receptors in the neuromuscular junction. Commonly used drugs in the class include atracurium, rocuronium, and vecuronium.

2.4.1.1 *Atracurium*

Atracurium is a commonly used non-depolarizing muscle relaxant. It is particularly useful in renal and hepatic failure, as a significant proportion of the drug is broken down spontaneously in the plasma and therefore does not depend on patient factors for termination of action.

Atracurium takes approximately 3 min to reach peak effect, and a single dose lasts for around 30 min.

Chemical name: 2,2'-{1,5-pentanediylbis[oxy(3-oxo-3,1-propanediyl)]}bis[1-(3,4-dimethoxybenzyl)-6,7-dimethoxy-2-methyl-1,2,3,4-tetrahydroisoquinolinium] dibenzenesulphonate.

Presentation: clear, colourless aqueous solution, commonly in ampoules containing 2.5 mL or 5 mL of solution with a concentration of 10 mg/mL. It must be kept in a refrigerator.

Dose: 0.5 mg/kg.

Respiratory: atracurium is a skeletal muscle relaxant that causes diaphragmatic and chest wall paralysis, thereby preventing spontaneous ventilation.

Cardiovascular: no direct cardiovascular effects.

Other: nil.

Side effects: atracurium is a potential trigger of anaphylaxis. It also triggers histamine release that can cause local cutaneous reactions, vasodilatation, hypotension, or bronchoconstriction.

Metabolism: 40% of the administered dose is broken down by either ester hydrolysis or by Hofmann elimination. The remainder is metabolized in the liver. Although atracurium has no active metabolites, metabolism yields laudanosine, which is potentially epileptogenic at high concentrations. This is very seldom significant in clinical practice.

2.4.1.2 *Rocuronium*

Rocuronium is a commonly used non-depolarizing muscle relaxant that is structurally related to vecuronium. Although, at lower doses, rocuronium has a slow onset time, similar to atracurium, it is sometimes used as an alternative to suxamethonium during RSIs. This is because, at high doses (>1 mg/kg), the onset time falls to around 60 s. Its long duration of action is potentially a hazard in the event of a failed intubation (see Section 7.2) so should only be used in this way under supervision.

Chemical name: 1-((2S,3S,5S,8R,9S,10S,13S,14S,16S,17R)-17-acetoxy-3-hydroxy-10,13-dimethyl-2-morpholinohexadecahydro-1H-cyclopenta[a]phenanthren-16-yl)-1-allylpyrrolidinium bromide.

Presentation: clear, colourless aqueous solution, commonly in ampoules containing 5 mL of solution with a concentration of 10 mg/mL. Must be kept in a refrigerator.

Dose: 0.6 mg/kg to 1.2 mg/kg.

Respiratory: rocuronium is a skeletal muscle relaxant that causes diaphragmatic and chest wall paralysis, thereby preventing spontaneous ventilation.

Cardiovascular: no direct cardiovascular effects.

Other: nil.

Side effects: potential trigger of anaphylaxis.

Metabolism: predominantly excreted unchanged via bile, with a small amount appearing in urine. It can accumulate in renal and hepatic failure, prolonging its action.

2.4.1.3 *Vecuronium*

Vecuronium is a non-depolarizing neuromuscular blocker, structurally related to rocuronium. It has minimal effects on the cardiovascular system and does not stimulate histamine release.

Onset time is comparable to atracurium and low-dose rocuronium.

Chemical name: [(2S,3S,5S,8R,9S,10S,13S,14S,16S,17S)-17-acetyloxy-10,13-dimethyl-16-(1-methyl-3,4,5,6-tetrahydro-2H-pyridin-1-yl)-2-(1-piperidyl)-2,3,4,5,6,7,8,9,11,12,14,15,16,17-tetradecahydro-1H-cyclopenta[a]phenanthren-3-yl] acetate.

Presentation: ampoules containing 10 mg of vecuronium as a white powder, for reconstitution in saline.

Dose: 0.1 mg/kg.

Respiratory: vecuronium is a skeletal muscle relaxant that causes diaphragmatic and chest wall paralysis, thereby preventing spontaneous ventilation.

Cardiovascular: nil.

Other: nil.

Side effects: vecuronium is a potential trigger of anaphylaxis.
Metabolism: hepatic metabolism to yield active metabolites. These metabolites have a very short half-life and are not normally clinically significant, although levels may accumulate in renal failure.

2.4.2 **Depolarizing neuromuscular blockade**

Only one depolarizing agent, suxamethonium, is in clinical use.

2.4.2.1 *Suxamethonium*

Suxamethonium is a depolarizing muscle relaxant, structurally related to acetylcholine. Suxamethonium use is essentially restricted to the RSI technique (see Section 5.2) and emergency management of laryngospasm (see Section 7.5.3). Suxamethonium can trigger MH (see Section 7.11).

Its mechanism of action results in visible generalized fasciculations, the offset of which indicates peak effect. It has a fast onset time (30–60 s) and a short duration of action (usually 5–8 min, although genetic variations can prolong this in some patients).

Chemical name: 2,2'-[(1,4-dioxobutane-1,4-diyl)bis(oxy)]bis(N,N,N-trimethylethanaminium).

Presentation: 2 mL ampoules of a clear and colourless solution containing 50 mg/mL. The drug must be kept in a refrigerator.

Dose: for RSI, the dose is 1.5 mg/kg. For emergency management of laryngospasm, a dose of 0.1 mg/kg is usually appropriate.

Respiratory: suxamethonium is a skeletal muscle relaxant that causes diaphragmatic and chest wall paralysis, thereby preventing spontaneous ventilation.

Cardiovascular: can cause bradycardia, particularly in children.

Other: suxamethonium increases intraocular pressure and ICP. Its use is associated with transient increases in serum potassium, which can precipitate an arrhythmia in patients with pre-existing hyperkalaemia.

Side effects: suxamethonium is a potential trigger of anaphylaxis. It triggers histamine release that can (rarely) cause cutaneous reactions, vasodilatation, hypotension, or bronchoconstriction. It is also a potential trigger for malignant hyperpyrexia. Suxamethonium use is associated with post-operative myalgia.

Metabolism: suxamethonium is broken down by plasma cholinesterase, with complete recovery by 12 min in most patients. Genetic variation in the cholinesterase enzyme can result in significantly prolonged duration of action. In homozygous patients (incidence 1:3000), suxamethonium can last for several hours, although heterozygotes (incidence 1:25) may experience milder prolongation of action of up to 10 min. See Section 7.6.

2.4.3 **Reversing neuromuscular blockade**

Neuromuscular blockade is routinely reversed, using a combined preparation of neostigmine and glycopyrrolate, but a new agent sugammadex can be used for the emergency reversal of neuromuscular block associated with vecuronium or rocuronium. Unlike neostigmine and glycopyrrolate, which cannot reverse complete blockade, sugammadex can be used successfully, even from full paralysis.

2.4.3.1 *Neostigmine and glycopyrrolate*

Neostigmine and glycopyrrolate (commonly referred to as 'reversal') are a compound preparation, useful for terminating the clinical effect of non-depolarizing neuromuscular blockade. It cannot be used to reverse complete neuromuscular blockade, and neuromuscular transmission must be assessed with a peripheral nerve stimulator prior to the dose being given to ensure timing is appropriate.

Neostigmine and glycopyrrolate cannot be used to reverse the effects of suxamethonium.

Neostigmine is a reversible inhibitor of acetylcholinesterase and works at both nicotinic and muscarinic acetylcholine receptors. Reduction in acetylcholine metabolism at the neuromuscular (nicotinic) receptors therefore increases acetylcholine concentration, allowing it to outcompete residual relaxant molecules and restore normal transmission. A generalized increase in acetylcholine concentration results in unwanted side effects, including bradycardia and bronchoconstriction, so the coadministration of an antimuscarinic (glycopyrrolate) minimizes this risk.

Chemical name: 3-{[(dimethylamino)carbonyl]oxy}-N,N,N-trimethylbenzenaminium; 3-(2-cyclopentyl-2-hydroxy-2-phenylacetoxy)-1,1-dimethylpyrrolidinium.

Presentation: presented in 1 mL ampoules containing a clear and colourless aqueous solution. Ampoules contain 2.5 mg of neostigmine and 500 micrograms of glycopyrrolate.

Dose: 0.02 mL/kg of solution is given to reverse partial neuromuscular blockade (two or more twitches demonstrated with peripheral nerve stimulator), repeatable up to a maximum of 2 mL.

Respiratory: muscarinic effects of neostigmine can result in bronchospasm.

Cardiovascular: antimuscarinic effects of glycopyrrolate often cause tachycardia.

Other: the antimuscarinic side effects of neostigmine and glycopyrrolate also include blurred vision, dry mouth, nausea, urinary retention, increased gastric and ureteric tone.

Side effects: increased gastrointestinal (GI) tone may threaten surgical anastamoses. Neostigmine will generally prolong effects of suxamethonium.

Metabolism: neostigmine is metabolized by acetylcholinesterase and by plasma cholinesterase. Some metabolism occurs in the liver. Although the kidney excretes the majority of the dose, a small amount is detectable in bile.

2.4.3.2 *Sugammadex*

Sugammadex is a novel agent designed for the reversal of rocuronium and vecuronium. Its mechanism of actions differs from neostigmine and glycopyrrolate, as, rather than inhibiting the metabolism of acetylcholine, sugammadex acts by selectively binding free drug molecules and preventing them from interacting with receptors. Sugammadex can be used for reversal of neuromuscular blockade, routinely at the end of a case or uniquely for emergency reversal of block with rocuronium from complete paralysis.

Presentation: 1, 2, or 5 mL ampoules containing 100 mg/mL of sugammadex.

Dose: for routine reversal of rocuronium or vecuronium, a dose of 2–4 mg/kg is given. For emergency reversal of rocuronium, 16 mg/kg is recommended.

Respiratory: nil, although patients should be monitored carefully for recurrence of neuromuscular blockade.

Cardiovascular: nil.

Other: sugammadex is a potential trigger of anaphylaxis.

Side effects: sugammadex may prolong activated partial thromboplastin time (aPTT) or prothrombin time (PT). This is not significant in patients receiving routine prophylactic low-molecular-weight heparin (LMWH), but caution should be exercised in patients who are therapeutically anticoagulated or have coagulopathies. Further doses of rocuronium or vecuronium should not be administered within 24 h of sugammadex.

Metabolism: sugammadex is excreted unchanged by the kidney and is not recommended in patients on dialysis or with severe renal failure (creatinine clearance <30 mL/min), although it can be given safely to those with mild to moderate renal impairment.

2.5 Sympathomimetic drugs and anticholinergics

Sympathomimetics are those drugs that have actions that mimic the activation of the sympathetic nervous system. Most commonly, they are used as vasoconstrictors or inotropes to maintain blood pressure during anaesthesia.

Anticholinergics are used in the treatment of symptomatic bradycardia and may be combined with drugs, such as neostigmine, for the reversal of non-depolarizing neuromuscular blockade. Anticholinergics may occasionally be used to decrease respiratory secretions and dry the oropharynx before airway interventions.

2.5.1 Sympathomimetic drugs

2.5.1.1 *Ephedrine*

Ephedrine is an indirectly acting sympathomimetic drug, with actions at α_1, β_1, and β_2 adrenergic receptors. It acts by increasing the release of noradrenaline from sympathetic nerve terminals and causes an increase in heart rate, stroke volume, and systemic vascular resistance.

Chemical name: (R*,S*)-2-(methylamino)-1-phenylpropan-1-ol.

Presentation: a clear and colourless aqueous solution containing 30 mg in 2 mL. Many anaesthetists dilute the 30 mg into 10 mL to yield 3 mg/mL.

Dose: generally given as 3–6 mg boluses, at intervals of approximately 5 min.

Respiratory: the β_2 effects of ephedrine cause bronchodilation.

Cardiovascular: the α_1 effects cause peripheral vasoconstriction, while β_1 effects result in increased stroke volume and heart rate.

Other: CNS stimulant, which may cause awareness at very light planes of anaesthesia.

Side effects: increased myocardial work may induce ischaemia in patients with coronary disease. Can provoke tachycardia, particularly in combination with other arrhythmogenic drugs.

Metabolism: ephedrine is excreted unchanged in urine, with only small quantities metabolized in the liver. Depletion of noradrenaline stores results in tachyphylaxis (as more drug is given, increasing doses are required to achieve the same effects).

2.5.1.2 *Metaraminol*

Metaraminol has both direct and indirect sympathomimetic effects, predominantly mediated via α_1 adrenoceptors, although it does retain some β_1 effects.

Chemical name: 3,β-dihydroxyamphetamine.

Presentation: 1 mL ampoule containing 10 mg metaraminol as a clear and colourless aqueous solution. It is commonly diluted into 10–20 mL of 0.9% saline for administration.

Dose: bolus doses of 500 micrograms are usually sufficient to correct moderate hypotension, although higher doses are occasionally required.

Respiratory: nil.

Cardiovascular: primarily metaraminol causes α-mediated vasoconstriction. Reflex bradycardia is not uncommon, and cardiac output can fall as a result of increased systemic vascular resistance.

Other: nil.

Side effects: nil.

Metabolism: mainly metabolized in the liver.

2.5.1.3 *Adrenaline*

Adrenaline is a potent inotrope, chronotrope, and bronchodilator, used for emergency support of the circulation in severe shock or cardiac arrest. It also has a crucial role in the treatment of anaphylaxis (see Section 7.7).

Chemical name: (R)-4-(1-hydroxy-2-(methylamino)ethyl)benzene-1,2-diol.

Presentation: adrenaline is available in a range of formulations, depending on the indication for its use. For circulatory support, it is supplied in 1 or 2 mL ampoules containing 1 mg/mL adrenaline for dilution. During cardiac arrest, it is presented in prefilled syringes containing 1 mg in 10 mL (i.e. a 1 in 10 000 solution). For use in anaphylaxis, it is supplied as 1 mg in 1 mL (i.e. a 1 in 1000 solution) in prefilled syringes.

Dose: by continuous infusion for circulatory support, adrenaline is given at a rate of 0.01–0.5 micrograms/kg/min. During cardiac arrest, IV bolus doses of 1 mg are required every 3–5 min (see Section 7.9). For anaphylaxis, the appropriate dose is 500 micrograms IM (see Section 7.7.1).

Respiratory: adrenaline is a profound bronchodilator and increases pulmonary vascular resistance.

Cardiovascular: the cardiovascular effects of adrenaline vary, depending on the dose administered. Predominantly β-effects (chronotropy, inotropy, and bronchodilation) are seen when given by low-dose infusion, although, when larger doses are given, α-effects (vasoconstriction) are more significant. These effects all increase myocardial work, which can precipitate cardiac ischaemia or arrhythmias.

Other: adrenaline increases plasma glucose, glucagon, and lactate concentration. Sympathetic stimulation also increases anaesthetic requirements and may even precipitate awareness in a lightly anaesthetized patient.

Side effects: nil.

Metabolism: metabolized by catecholamine-O-methyl transferase and monoamine oxidase. Great care should be used if adrenaline is required in a patient taking monoamine oxidase-inhibitor (MAO-I) therapy.

2.5.2 **Anticholinergic drugs**

2.5.2.1 *Atropine*

Atropine is a competitive antagonist at muscarinic acetylcholine receptors and is primarily used in the treatment of symptomatic bradycardia.

Chemical name: (RS)-(8-methyl-8-azabicyclo[3.2.1]oct-3-yl) 3-hydroxy-2-phenylpropanoate.

Presentation: available in prefilled syringes containing 100–600 micrograms/mL. Also available in 1 mL ampoules containing 600 micrograms/mL.

Dose: for emergency treatment of symptomatic bradycardia, 500 micrograms of atropine are given every 5 min, until the heart rate improves or a maximum of 3 mg is reached (see Section 7.10.2). Routine treatment of bradycardia is usually given with initial IV boluses of 300 micrograms.

Respiratory: atropine is a bronchodilator and reduces respiratory secretions.

Cardiac: atropine raises heart rate and may result in tachycardia.

Other: atropine crosses the blood–brain barrier so can cause confusion, particularly in the elderly.

Side effects: in common with other anticholinergics, atropine can cause constipation, urinary retention, blurred vision, photophobia, and dry mouth.

Metabolism: atropine undergoes hepatic metabolism and is excreted in urine.

2.5.2.2 *Glycopyrrolate*

Glycopyrrolate has similar effects to atropine, but it differs slightly in structure, giving it a slightly slower onset and longer duration of action. The molecule is large and permanently charged, which prevents it from crossing the blood–brain barrier, so, unlike atropine, glycopyrrolate does not cause confusion.

It is usually used in routine perioperative treatment of bradycardia and occasionally also to reduce respiratory secretions prior to airway instrumentation. It is also commonly combined with neostigmine for reversal of neuromuscular blockade (see Section 2.4.3.1) where its antimuscarinic actions prevent unwanted parasympathetic responses.

Chemical name: 3-(2-cyclopentyl-2-hydroxy-2-phenylacetoxy)-1,1-dimethylpyrrolidinium.

Presentation: supplied in 1 or 3 mL ampoules, containing 200 micrograms/mL.

Dose: 200–400 micrograms.

Respiratory: glycopyrrolate causes bronchodilation and reduced respiratory secretions.

Cardiac: glycopyrrolate raises heart rate, although probably to a lesser degree than atropine.

Other: nil.

Side effects: in common with other anticholinergics, glycopyrrolate can cause constipation, urinary retention, blurred vision, photophobia, and dry mouth.

Metabolism: glycopyrrolate is predominantly excreted unchanged in urine, with only a small proportion metabolized in the liver.

2.6 Analgesics

Analgesics are amongst the commonest drugs administered perioperatively, and the anaesthetist is responsible for providing an analgesic plan for the patient in the immediate post-operative phase. The anaesthetist is also often the first point of contact for ward staff seeking analgesic advice.

Analgesia is generally prescribed according to the World Health Organization (WHO) analgesic ladder. For more information about post-operative planning, see Section 3.4.4.

2.6.1 Paracetamol

Paracetamol is usually the first drug given to treat pain and is a useful component of multimodal analgesic therapy where it is given in combination with other classes of analgesic drugs. Side effects and allergies are rare, although it can be toxic when given in inappropriate doses. Care should be taken in children and chronically ill or malnourished adults that doses are appropriate to the patient's weight.

Chemical name: N-(4-hydroxyphenyl)ethanamide.

Presentation: available orally as: tablets, dispersible tablets, or capsules (120 mg or 500 mg); or as oral suspensions of 120 mg/5 mL and 250 mg/5 mL. For rectal administration, paracetamol is presented as suppositories of 60 mg, 125 mg, 250 mg, 500 mg, and 1 g. For IV administration, it is presented as a clear, colourless aqueous solution containing 10 mg/mL in volumes of 50 mL or 100 mL.

Dose: 20 mg/kg by oral or rectal route (maximum 1 g/24 h); 15 mg/kg if given IV (maximum 1 g/24 h); interval 4–6 hourly.

Respiratory: no effects.

Cardiovascular: paracetamol delivered by IV infusion can result in hypotension or tachycardia.

Other: nil.

Side effects: at therapeutic doses, side effects to paracetamol are extremely rare, although occasionally paracetamol use can result in a variety of haematological disorders.

Metabolism: metabolism is primarily hepatic, by a combination of glucuronidation, sulfation, and N-hydroxylation. Although N-hydroxylation accounts for only 15% of paracetamol metabolism, it yields a toxic metabolite N-acetyl-p-benzo-quinoneimine (NAPQI). NAPQI is normally rapidly conjugated with glutathione, rendering it non-toxic. This pathway is easily saturated in overdose, and NAPQI is responsible for hepatotoxicity after paracetamol overdose. Treatment with N-acetyl-cysteine replenishes glutathione stores. The decision to treat is based on paracetamol levels and is guided by published nomograms.

2.6.2 **Non-steroidal anti-inflammatory drugs**

Non-steroidal anti-inflammatory drugs (NSAIDs) are very useful analgesics for perioperative use, although side effects mean that care must be taken to ensure prescribing is appropriate.

All NSAIDs possess antiplatelet actions and can be associated with post-operative bleeding. They are frequently and safely prescribed after most general surgical operations, but caution should be exercised after surgery where bleeding is a particular risk, including neurosurgery, ear, nose, and throat (ENT) or maxillo-facial surgery, and after some orthopaedic operations. If in doubt, seek the advice of senior colleagues. There has also been recent evidence of prolonged NSAID use increasing the risk of thrombotic events (including myocardial infarction and stroke), so NSAID use should be for the shortest appropriate duration.

NSAIDs share common absolute contraindications:

- Active GI bleeding or past history, or peptic ulcer disease
- Renal impairment
- Heart failure
- Known allergy or known NSAID-sensitive asthma
- Third trimester of pregnancy.

NSAIDs should be used with caution in the following groups:

- Age >65
- Asthmatics
- Diabetes
- Uncontrolled hypertension
- Ischaemic heart disease
- Peripheral vascular disease

- Inflammatory bowel disease
- First or second trimester of pregnancy.

2.6.2.1 *Ibuprofen*

Ibuprofen is a frequently prescribed NSAID and is derived from propionic acid. It has the lowest incidence of side effects of the most commonly used NSAIDs. Although IV preparations are available in some European countries and Australasia, in the UK, ibuprofen is only available for oral administration.

Chemical name: (RS)-2-(4-(2-methylpropyl)phenyl)propanoic acid.

Presentation: tablets or capsules (200 mg or 400 mg), or as an oral suspension with a concentration of 100 mg/5 mL.

Dose: 300–400 mg, 3–4 times a day, up to a maximum of 2.4 g/24 h.

Respiratory: non-selective inhibition of cyclo-oxygenase (COX) can cause bronchoconstriction in susceptible individuals, but only a small proportion (probably fewer than 20%) of asthmatics are at risk.

Cardiovascular: nil.

Other: nil.

Side effects: ibuprofen may be associated with increased surgical bleeding, although this is infrequently a clinical problem. All NSAIDs may increase the risk of cardiovascular events after prolonged use. They are also associated with peptic ulceration, GI bleeding, and deranged renal function. Fluid retention may precipitate heart failure in at-risk patients.

Metabolism: metabolized by the liver to inactive metabolites that are excreted in the urine.

2.6.2.2 *Diclofenac*

Diclofenac is derived from phenylacetic acid. One advantage diclofenac possesses over ibuprofen is that it is available for a wider range of routes, including IV and PR.

Chemical name: 2-(2-(2,6-dichlorophenylamino)phenyl)acetic acid.

Presentation: available orally as tablets or dispersible tablets (25 mg or 50 mg). For rectal administration, presented as suppositories of 12.5 mg, 25 mg, 50 mg, 100 mg, and 1 g. For IV administration, presented as a clear, colourless aqueous solution containing 75 mg of diclofenac in 3 mL. It should be diluted and infused over 30 min.

Dose: 75–150 mg/day in two or three divided doses, to a maximum of 150 mg/24 h.

Respiratory: non-selective inhibition of COX can cause bronchoconstriction in susceptible individuals, but only a small proportion (probably fewer than 20%) of asthmatics are at risk.

Cardiovascular: nil.

Other: nil.

Side effects: diclofenac may be associated with increased surgical bleeding, although this is infrequently a clinical problem. All NSAIDs may increase the risk of cardiovascular events after prolonged use. They are also associated with peptic ulceration, GI bleeding, and deranged renal function. Fluid retention may precipitate heart failure in at-risk patients.

Metabolism: metabolized by the liver to inactive metabolites that are excreted in the urine.

2.6.3 **Opioids**

Opioids are commonly used throughout the perioperative period. It should be noted that there is a difference between the terms opiate and opioid; 'opiate' specifically refers to naturally occurring narcotic agents derived from the opium poppy *Papaver somniferum*. The term opioid refers to all drugs, natural and synthetic, that are agonists at opioid receptors.

2.6.3.1 *Codeine phosphate*

Codeine phosphate is around ten times less potent than morphine but is a useful drug when coadministered with simple analgesics and NSAIDs in the treatment of moderate to severe pain. Codeine is available for oral and IM use.

Chemical name: (5α,6α)-7,8-didehydro-4,5-epoxy-3-methoxy-17-methylmorphinan-6-ol.

Presentation: for oral use, codeine is presented as 15 mg, 30 mg, and 60 mg tablets, or in syrup form containing 25 mg/mL. The IM preparation contains 60 mg/mL.

Dose: 30–60 mg, 4–6 hourly, up to a maximum of 240 mg/24 h.

Respiratory: μ receptor activation causes hypoventilation, predominantly through a reduction in respiratory rate. Respiratory centre sensitivity to CO_2 falls. Antitussive effects.

Cardiovascular: codeine may cause bradycardia and hypotension, associated with reduced sympathetic tone. Codeine has no direct myocardial effects.

Other: GI effects of codeine include decreased gastric emptying, constipation, nausea, and vomiting. It is also sedative, particularly with increasing dose.

Side effects: codeine can be associated with histamine release. Itch is also a feature but is probably not histamine-related.

Metabolism: codeine undergoes hepatic metabolism, predominantly via 6-hydroxyl glucuronidation. Ten to 20% undergoes N-demethylation to norcodeine, and 15% via O-demethylation to morphine (the only codeine metabolite with significant opioid receptor activity). Ten per cent of the UK population lack this enzyme to metabolize codeine to morphine and therefore experience a lesser analgesic effect.

2.6.3.2 *Fentanyl*[CD]

Fentanyl is a synthetic opioid, with approximately ten times the potency of morphine, and faster onset and offset. Duration of action after a single bolus is around 30 min. Fentanyl is a controlled drug.

Fentanyl can also be given by continuous infusion for sedation purposes or used in patient-controlled analgesia (PCA) regimens.

Fentanyl is most commonly used IV, but high lipid solubility makes it suitable for transdermal, subcutaneous, or buccal administration; patches and lollipops are available for palliative and chronic pain use. It is also commonly used in central neuraxial blockade.

Chemical name: N-(1-(2-phenylethyl)-4-piperidinyl)-N-phenylpropanamide.

Presentation: fentanyl is most commonly encountered as a clear, colourless aqueous solution containing 50 micrograms/mL in 2 mL ampoules. Transdermal patches are generally prescribed on a dose-per-hour basis and are available with release rates of 25–100 micrograms/h. Patches generally last for 72 h. Lollipops contain 200–1600 micrograms, but slow absorption means patches and lollipops are not suitable for treatment of acute pain.

Dose: for treatment of acute pain or induction of anaesthesia, doses of up to 1 microgram/kg are usually appropriate. Doses of 12–50 micrograms are commonly used in spinal anaesthesia when combined with local anaesthetic (LA) agents.

Respiratory: μ receptor activation causes hypoventilation, predominantly through a reduction in respiratory rate. Respiratory centre sensitivity to CO_2 falls. Fentanyl has antitussive effects.

Cardiovascular: fentanyl causes bradycardia and hypotension, associated with reduced sympathetic tone. Fentanyl has no direct myocardial effects.

Other: GI effects of fentanyl include decreased gastric emptying, constipation, and nausea and vomiting. It is sedative, particularly with increasing dose.

Side effects: fentanyl use can be associated with histamine release. Itch is also a feature but is probably not histamine-related.

Metabolism: fentanyl is metabolized in the liver to yield inactive metabolites. It is generally considered safer in renal failure than morphine.

2.6.3.3 *Morphine sulfate*[CD]

Morphine sulfate is the reference opioid against which others are compared. It is naturally occurring, and a wide variety of formulations are available, suitable for IV, IM, PR, and oral use. Although it can be used subcutaneously, morphine is not very lipid-soluble, therefore absorption is variable. Preservative-free morphine formulations are occasionally used in central neuraxial blockade. Most formulations of morphine are controlled, although some low-strength oral solutions are not.

Chemical name: (5α,6α)-7,8-didehydro-4,5-epoxy-17-methylmorphinan-3,6-diol.

Presentation: a variety of strengths and formulations are available, but the most commonly available preparation in theatre is a 1 mL ampoule containing 10 mg/mL of morphine.

Dose: for treatment of acute pain, doses of up to 100 micrograms/kg are generally appropriate. Oral doses are approximately twice the equivalent IV bolus and are repeatable after 2 h.

Respiratory: μ receptor activation causes hypoventilation, predominantly through reduction in respiratory rate. Respiratory centre sensitivity to CO_2 falls. Morphine has antitussive effects.

Cardiovascular: morphine causes bradycardia and hypotension, associated with reduced sympathetic tone. Morphine has no direct myocardial effects.

Other: the GI effects of morphine include decreased gastric emptying, constipation, and nausea and vomiting. It is sedative, particularly with increasing dose.

Side effects: morphine can be associated with histamine release. Itch is a feature but is probably not histamine-related.

Metabolism: morphine undergoes hepatic metabolism to morphine-3-glucuronide and morphine-6-glucuronide. Morphine-6-glucuronide is 13 times more potent than morphine and is excreted by the kidney. Morphine is therefore used with caution in patients with renal failure.

2.7 Antiemetics

PONV is a common complication of general anaesthesia and is a frequent cause of unexpected admission after day-case surgery. Certain identifiable patient groups are at increased risk from PONV:

- Females
- Non-smokers
- Past history of PONV
- Likely need for post-operative opioids
- High-risk surgery (squint surgery, some ENT techniques).

Patients with no risk factors do not generally require antiemetic prophylaxis. Patients with a single factor may also not require any treatment, but the more risk factors there are, the more appropriate prophylaxis would become. It may be appropriate in patients at particularly high risk to use a total intravenous anaesthesia (TIVA) technique, as this avoids exposure to inhalational anaesthetics entirely and capitalizes on the antiemetic properties of propofol.

2.7.1 Steroids

Antiemetic properties of steroids have been noted in anaesthetics, oncology, and palliative care, but the mechanism of action is unclear. Single doses of dexamethasone 4–8 mg given at induction have been used successfully in PONV prophylaxis.

2.7.1.1 *Dexamethasone*

Dexamethasone is a potent synthetic glucocorticoid. It is 27 times more potent than cortisol and seven times more potent than prednisolone.

Chemical name: (8S,9R,10S,11S,13S,14S,16R,17R)-9-fluoro-11,17-dihydroxy-17-(2-hydroxyacetyl)-10,13,16-trimethyl-6,7,8,9,10,11,12,13,14,15,16,17-dodecahydro-3H-cyclopenta[a]phenanthren-3-one.

Presentation: 1 or 2 mL ampoules of clear and colourless aqueous solution containing 4 mg/mL. Some formulations are presented in brown glass ampoules to protect the contents from light.

Dose: a single IV dose of 4–8 mg at induction is indicated for PONV prophylaxis.

Respiratory: nil.

Cardiovascular: nil.

Other: nil.

Side effects: if given prior to induction, dexamethasone can provoke abnormal perineal sensations. Single doses do not generally cause significant renal or GI effects but may worsen glycaemic control in diabetics.

Metabolism: dexamethasone is metabolized in the liver.

2.7.2 **Histamine antagonists**

H_1 receptor antagonists are of use in the prophylaxis and treatment of PONV. Although the exact site of action is unclear, it is postulated that they act on receptors in the chemoreceptor trigger zone (CTZ). H_2 antagonists (such as ranitidine) do not possess antiemetic properties.

2.7.2.1 *Cyclizine*

Cyclizine acts predominantly via competitive antagonism at H_1 receptors, but the drug also possesses central anticholinergic effects that may contribute both to antiemetic and adverse effects. Cyclizine is available for oral, IV, and IM use.

Chemical name: 1-benzhydryl-4-methyl-piperazine.

Presentation: for oral use, cyclizine is presented as 50 mg tablets. For IV or IM use, it is presented as a clear, colourless aqueous solution of 50 mg/mL in 1 mL ampoules.

Dose: 50 mg 8-hourly, by any route, to a maximum of 150 mg/24 h.

Respiratory: nil.

Cardiovascular: the anticholinergic effect of cyclizine can result in tachycardia, especially after IV dose.

Other: the central anticholinergic effects can cause confusion or sedation, especially in the elderly. Increases lower oesophageal sphincter tone.

Side effects: anticholinergic effects, including dry eyes, dry mouth, and blurred vision.

Metabolism: cyclizine is metabolized to norcyclizine in the liver by N-demethylation.

2.7.3 **Dopamine antagonists**

The CTZ contains a large concentration of D_2 dopaminergic receptors. A number of drugs with antiemetic properties act through dopaminergic receptors, including metoclopramide, prochlorperazine, and chlorpromazine.

Although these drugs have some useful antiemetic properties; their use can be limited by significant extrapyramidal side effects, and they do not usually form the first line of antiemetic therapy. The prokinetic properties of metoclopramide mean some anaesthetists use it prior to RSI (see Section 5.2).

2.7.3.1 *Metoclopramide*

Metoclopramide is a centrally acting D_2 receptor antagonist with some peripheral dopaminergic and cholinergic effects. It is occasionally used as a prokinetic agent, increasing gastric emptying. Metoclopramide is available for IV, IM, and oral use.

Chemical name: 4-amino-5-chloro-N-(2-(diethylamino)ethyl)-2-methoxybenzamide.

Presentation: for oral use; is presented as 10 mg tablets. A solution for parenteral use is available, containing 5 mg/mL in 2 mL ampoules.

Dose: 10 mg 8-hourly, to a maximum of 30 mg/24 h.

Respiratory: nil.

Cardiovascular: metoclopramide can cause tachy- or bradycardia, or hypotension after rapid IV administration.

Other: increases lower oesophageal sphincter tone and increases gastric emptying.

Side effects: sedation or extrapyramidal effects can occur up to 72 h after a metoclopramide dose. Side effects are more common in young women.

Metabolism: predominantly metabolized in the liver.

2.7.4 **Serotonin antagonists**

In addition to dopaminergic receptors, the vomiting centre and CTZ are also richly supplied with 5-HT_3 receptors. Only two serotonin antagonists are available in the UK for the treatment of PONV: ondansetron and granisetron.

2.7.4.1 *Ondansetron*

Ondansetron is a highly specific 5-HT_3 receptor antagonist. It has both central and peripheral actions, downregulating signals from the vomiting centre and CTZ. Ondansetron is available for oral, IM, or IV use.

Chemical name: (RS)-9-methyl-3-[(2-methyl-1H-imidazol-1-yl)methyl]-2,3-dihydro-1H-carbazol-4(9H)-one.

Presentation: presented as tablets (4 mg) or as an oral solution (4 mg/5 mL). For IV or IM use, it is presented as a clear, colourless aqueous solution of 2 mg/mL in 2 mL ampoules.

Dose: 4 mg as a single IV dose, repeatable 8-hourly for 24 h.

Respiratory: nil.

Cardiovascular: nil.

Other: nil.

Side effects: the drug is generally well tolerated but can be associated with constipation and headaches.

Metabolism: extensively metabolized in the liver. Doses must be reduced in liver failure but do not need to be altered in renal impairment.

2.8 Local anaesthetics

LAs are commonly used perioperatively, both by surgeons and anaesthetists. They are useful for local infiltration of wound sites, peripheral nerve blocks, or central neuraxial blockade (see Section 6.2).

All LAs share a common mechanism of action, blocking fast sodium channels and therefore preventing the propagation of action potentials along the nerve fibre.

LAs can be combined with vasoconstrictors to improve haemostasis and, in some cases, to prolong their duration of action. If using such a preparation, care should be taken not to inject into body extremities, as vasoconstriction can disrupt blood supply and result in necrosis.

The clinical effects of LAs are pH-dependent. They work poorly in acidic conditions so are not effective in local infiltration of infected tissue. Conversely, raising pH by adding 8.4% sodium bicarbonate can speed the onset of some LA agents.

Care must be taken to give appropriate doses of LAs, as all LAs can be toxic at high doses (see Section 7.8).

2.8.1 **Lidocaine**

Lidocaine is a relatively short-acting LA that can be used for local infiltration or nerve blocks. It can also be used epidurally, although spinal lidocaine is seldom used due to transient neurological symptoms occurring during recovery.

Mixtures of lidocaine and prilocaine, presented as EMLA® cream, can be used for topical anaesthesia prior to cannulation.

Chemical name: 2-(diethylamino)-N-(2,6-dimethylphenyl)acetamide.

Presentation: a clear, colourless aqueous solution of either 1 or 2% (10 or 20 mg/mL). Ampoules are available in a variety of sizes, from 1 mL to 10 mL, and are available with or without 1:200 000 adrenaline.

Dose: the maximum safe dose of lidocaine is 3 mg/kg (or 7 mg/kg if mixed with 1:200 000 adrenaline).

Respiratory: there are no direct effects on the respiratory system, but regional blocks may affect respiratory mechanics by inhibition of motor nerves.

Cardiac: blockade of cardiac sodium channels can result in dangerous arrhythmias. Historically, lidocaine had a specialist role in the treatment of some ventricular arrhythmias, but other anti-arrhythmic agents, such as amiodarone, have largely supplanted this. If an adrenaline-containing solution is used, tachycardia may be noted.

Other: toxic doses can cause central neurological effects, including altered consciousness and seizures. Clinical effects depend on the site of injection and dose given.

Side effects: toxic effects as noted in 'Other'.

Metabolism: hepatic metabolism, which may be prolonged in liver or cardiac failure.

2.8.2 **Bupivacaine**

Bupivacaine is one of the most commonly used LA drugs. It is highly protein-bound, giving a longer duration of action than lidocaine, but this also means it is potentially more hazardous in toxic doses, since it takes more time for effects to subside.

Bupivacaine is a racemic mixture of two enantiomers and a newer formulation (levobupivacaine), which contains only the S-enantiomer, is theoretically less toxic in overdose.

Although bupivacaine with adrenaline mixtures are available, the high protein-binding of bupivacaine means neither the duration of action nor the systemic absorption is significantly altered by the presence of the vasoconstrictor. These formulations are popular with surgeons, as vasoconstriction aids haemostasis, but they do not alter the maximum permitted dose.

A hyperbaric solution of bupivacaine (often referred to as 'heavy' bupivacaine) is available for spinal injection (see Section 6.2.2). This solution also contains 8% glucose, which raises the specific gravity of the solution. As the solution is denser than the cerebrospinal fluid (CSF) into which it is injected, the drug sinks predictably. By positioning the patient carefully on the bed, the spread of the LA, and therefore the extent of the clinical effect, can be controlled. Non-glucose-containing solutions are either of equal density (isobaric) or slightly lower than CSF (hypobaric) and therefore can spread through CSF somewhat less predictably.

Chemical name: (RS)-1-butyl-N-(2,6-dimethylphenyl)piperidine-2-carboxamide.

Presentation: available in 0.25% or 0.5% solutions (2.5 mg/mL or 5 mg/mL) in 10 mL ampoules, with or without 1:200 000 adrenaline. Heavy bupivacaine is available in 4 mL ampoules containing 0.5% (5 mg/mL) bupivacaine and 80 mg/mL glucose. Infusion bags for epidural use are available, generally with concentrations of around 0.1% (1 mg/mL). These infusions may also contain an opioid such as fentanyl.

Dose: the maximum permitted dose is 2 mg/kg, with or without adrenaline.

Respiratory: bupivacaine has no direct effects on the respiratory system, but regional blocks may affect respiratory mechanics by inhibition of motor nerves.

Cardiac: cardiac toxicity with bupivacaine is significant and long-lasting. Care must be taken at all times that doses are appropriate and the risk of intravascular injection is minimized. Adrenaline-containing solutions may cause tachycardia.

Other: toxic doses can cause central neurological effects, including altered consciousness and seizures. Clinical effects depend on the site of injection and dose given.

Side effects: toxic effects as noted in 'Other'.

Metabolism: metabolized in the liver.

2.9 Self-assessment questions

Answer either true or false for each of the following questions. The answers can be found in Appendix 2.

1. The following drugs can be used as induction agents:
   A. Isoflurane
   B. Ephedrine
   C. Atracurium
   D. Sodium thiopental
   E. Sevoflurane

2. Which of the following are associated with the use of propofol?
   A. Vasodilation
   B. Antiemesis
   C. Tissue damage on extravasation
   D. Pain on IV injection
   E. Analgesia

3. Concerning sodium thiopental:
   A. The drug is supplied as a clear, colourless aqueous solution
   B. Induction doses of 3–7 mg/kg may be required
   C. Thiopental reduces ICP
   D. Thiopental is rapidly metabolized when given by IV infusion
   E. The drug is contraindicated in patients with porphyria

4. Which of the following are suitable for the maintenance of general anaesthesia?
   A. Sodium thiopental
   B. Propofol
   C. Desflurane
   D. Sevoflurane
   E. Midazolam

5. Concerning MAC:
   A. The MAC of desflurane is 5.75%
   B. The MAC of sevoflurane is 2.00%
   C. The MAC of isoflurane is 1.10%
   D. MAC is defined in terms of conscious level
   E. MAC is reduced in the presence of nitrous oxide

6. Concerning the colour coding of vaporizers:

   A. A yellow vaporizer contains sevoflurane
   B. A red vaporizer contains desflurane
   C. A blue vaporizer contains nitrous oxide
   D. A purple vaporizer contains isoflurane
   E. An orange vaporizer contains oxygen

7. Which of the following agents may trigger MH in a susceptible individual?

   A. Propofol
   B. Suxamethonium
   C. Sodium thiopental
   D. Atracurium
   E. Desflurane

8. Neostigmine and glycopyrrolate can be used to reverse the effects of which of these drugs?

   A. Propofol
   B. Rocuronium
   C. Fentanyl
   D. Suxamethonium
   E. Mivacurium

9. Which of the following drugs would be expected to raise heart rate?

   A. Metaraminol
   B. Ephedrine
   C. Glycopyrrolate
   D. Propofol
   E. Cyclizine

10. Which of the following statements about morphine are true?

   A. Morphine is an agonist at μ, κ, and δ receptors
   B. Morphine is a synthetic opioid
   C. All presentations of morphine are controlled drugs
   D. Morphine is the drug of choice when administering opioids by the subcutaneous route
   E. An oral morphine dose of 20 mg is approximately equivalent to an IV dose of 10 mg

Chapter 3

Planning for general anaesthesia

3.1 Introduction

Safe delivery of anaesthesia requires careful planning. Ideally, all patients should be assessed prior to their arrival in theatre so the anaesthetic team can have the appropriate range of drugs and equipment ready. All members of the anaesthetic team should be briefed before the patient arrives.

3.2 Anaesthetic assessment

All patients should be assessed prior to coming to theatre. Ideally, the anaesthetist who will be looking after the patient should be the one to perform the assessment; however, in practice, this is not always possible.

Junior anaesthetists (particularly those in their first few months of training) will not be expected to anaesthetize a patient with significant comorbidities without the assistance of a senior colleague, but it is important to be able to identify those patients with more complex needs.

3.2.1 The anaesthetic history

Although individual anaesthetists develop their own way of conducting this assessment, there are essential pieces of information that must be taken in order to make the assessment complete. These details are then recorded on a suitable anaesthetic chart (see Fig 3.1). The assessment is essentially identical, regardless of the anaesthetic technique planned.

3.2.1.1 *Previous anaesthetic history*

Identify if a patient has had a general anaesthetic before, and, if so, determine if there were any difficulties. Certain problems may be recurrent, e.g. MH (see Section 7.11) or suxamethonium apnoea (see Section 7.6). Patients should also have been made aware of episodes of anaphylaxis (see Section 7.7) or airway difficulties in previous anaesthetics (see Sections 7.2 and 7.5). Note that a previous anaesthetic that went 'as planned' does not preclude difficulties in the future.

If a patient has previously undergone general anaesthesia, determine if they suffered PONV. A previous episode of PONV implies increased risk of recurrence with future anaesthetics (see Section 2.7).

Department of Anaesthetics

Preoperative notes and signed consent

Hospital number ______	Age	Weight:	ASA:
Surname ______		NCEPOD:	
First name ______	M/F	L S U E	

Procedure(s) proposed:

Anaesthetist's preoperative assessment by Dr ______ (date: / / time:)

BP
Hb
Hbs
K+ (3.5–5.0 mmol/L)
Creatinine (70–154micromol/L
Blood ordered
Blood transfusion Y / N

Technique proposed: (Please also indicate any technique(s) to which the patient does not agree)

I confirm that I have explained to the patient/parent(s)/guardian(s)* the type of anaesthesia/analgesia (general/regional/sedation/rectal/etc.) proposed in terms which in my judgement are suited to the understanding of the patient and/or one of the parents or guardians of the patient.

______ Signature

______ Name & grade of anaesthetist (PRINTED)

For attention of ward staff: (further investigations, fasting, continue/omit current medication, etc.)

ALL ORDERS/INFORMATION REGARDING MEDICATION & FLUIDS MUST BE ENTERED ON PATIENT'S DRUG PRESCRIPTION & ADMINISTRATION RECORD

Fig 3.1 An example of the front page of an anaesthetic chart.

Reproduced with kind permission from Oxford University Hospitals NHS Trust.

3.2.1.2 *Take a brief medical history*

Any comorbidity can affect the conduct or safety of anaesthesia. Comorbidities should be systematically identified, and the anaesthetist must gain an impression of the severity, current treatment, and the extent to which patients are limited by their disease.

Although the following list is by no means exhaustive, some of the more common important conditions to identify include:

1. **Cardiac:** ischaemic heart disease, cardiac failure, and dysrhythmias.
   All of these conditions increase the risk of perioperative morbidity. It is important to note what provokes symptoms, how well controlled symptoms are, and whether there has been any recent change. Note also if any anticoagulant or antiplatelet therapy is ongoing and if any cardiac stents, pacemakers, or other devices are present.

2. **Respiratory:** asthma, chronic obstructive airways disease (COAD), restrictive lung diseases.
   Anaesthesia has significant effects on the respiratory system, and patients with respiratory disease can present the anaesthetist with significant difficulties. Note how well symptoms are controlled and what therapy is currently used. Record if asthmatic patients have ever been admitted and/or ventilated previously. Recent steroid therapy may indicate adrenal suppression. The response of asthmatic patients to NSAIDs is particularly important.

3. **Metabolic:** diabetes (type I or type II), obesity.
   Steps must be taken to minimize disruption to the patient's normal regimen and to monitor capillary glucose regularly. Evidence of end-organ damage should be noted. Ideally, diabetic patients should be first on the operating list to minimize fasting time. Autonomic neuropathy may result in haemodynamic instability on induction, and gastric emptying may be prolonged. Other metabolic conditions may have a significant impact, e.g. a range of anaesthetic drugs is contraindicated in porphyria. Long-standing diabetes and obesity may both suggest a difficult intubation, cardiac comorbidities, and hypertension.

4. **Musculoskeletal:** rheumatoid arthritis, ankylosing spondylitis.
   Patients with musculoskeletal or connective tissue diseases often have multisystem involvement that requires careful assessment. Rheumatoid arthritis can affect the heart, lungs, kidneys, and peripheral nervous system, in addition to the obvious musculoskeletal involvement. Such patients may also present airway difficulties related to problems with positioning, unstable cervical spines, or limitations in mouth opening. Steroid therapy or immunosuppressive drugs are also relevant.

5. **Neurological:** multiple sclerosis, spinal abnormalities, myasthenia gravis, epilepsy.
   Neurological conditions can have variable effects, depending on the disease process. Myasthenia gravis patients or those with spinal cord injuries may have abnormal responses to muscle relaxants and may require elective ventilation post-operatively. Patients with head injuries or intracranial mass lesions may be at risk from increased ICP, and special precautions must be taken at each stage of the anaesthetic to protect them. The old volatile anaesthetic agent enflurane was pro-epileptogenic and could induce seizures in those at risk. Congenital or acquired spinal abnormalities (including previous surgery) are particularly relevant if a spinal or epidural technique is planned.

6. **Renal:** renal failure or impairment.

Renal failure or impairment affects the metabolism and distribution of a number of anaesthetic drugs. Patients on dialysis are often fluid-restricted and (depending on when they last received dialysis) may be volume-deplete, euvolaemic, or fluid-overloaded. Care must be taken to avoid nephrotoxic agents in patients with residual renal function. Transplanted patients will be on a range of immunosuppressive therapies and require specialist input.

3.2.1.3 *Drug treatment and allergies*

It is important to note what medications a patient is receiving. It is also often worthwhile asking about any treatments that have been recently discontinued, especially steroid therapy.

It may be relevant to establish if a patient has used any recreational substances or alcohol.

Any allergies, and the nature of any reaction, should be recorded.

3.2.1.4 *Smoking history*

All patients should be asked if they are current or ex-smokers. Not only is smoking a risk factor for respiratory and cardiovascular disease, but smoking also increases respiratory mucus production and may make the airway more irritable at induction or emergence. The anaesthetist should be aware of this increased risk and be vigilant for events such as laryngospasm (see Section 7.5.3). The increased risk from smoking returns to normal after around 6 weeks of abstinence.

3.2.1.5 *Fasting state*

The time a patient last ate and drank should be recorded. A patient is considered fasted (i.e. does not require an RSI) if:

- No solid food or milk-containing fluid has been consumed within the last 6 h
- No clear fluids have been consumed within the last 2 h.

There are some circumstances where these timings may not be reliable. Pain, trauma, some drugs (opioids, in particular), some pathologies (including diabetic autonomic neuropathy and surgical conditions) all slow gastric emptying, and an RSI may still be appropriate, even if the last intake was some time ago. Patients with symptomatic gastro-oesophageal reflux may also be at additional risk and can require RSI, even when apparently fasted.

3.2.1.6 *Dentition*

The state of the patient's dentition should be recorded. Any loose teeth or crowns are at risk of damage during anaesthesia, and the edentulous patient may be difficult to mask-ventilate.

3.2.2 **Airway assessment**

All patients should have a careful airway assessment conducted.

Two crucial questions must be answered after an airway assessment. First, the anaesthetist must identify patients in whom face mask ventilation may be difficult. This could include the obese, bearded patients, those with significant facial trauma or deformity, and edentulous patients.

Second, the anaesthetist must attempt to predict patients at risk of a difficult intubation. This assessment should be made, regardless of whether intubation is planned.

Adequate airway assessment comprises three different examinations: Mallampati score, measurement of thyromental distance, and assessment of jaw protrusion. In isolation, none of the tests have high predictive value; however, in combination, they predict many difficult intubations.

A difficult airway is one where a trained anaesthetist experiences problems performing mask ventilation, performing intubation, or both.

3.2.2.1 *Mallampati score*

This is scored against a four-point scale, illustrated in Fig 3.2:

- **Grade I:** the tonsils, uvula, soft palate, and hard palate are visible. This is reassuring and generally associated with good view at laryngoscopy
- **Grade II:** the soft palate and hard palate are visible, but the lower parts of the tonsils and uvula are obscured. This is usually reassuring
- **Grade III:** the soft and hard palate are visible, but only the base of the uvula can be seen. This can be associated with difficult views at direct laryngoscopy
- **Grade IV:** only the hard palate is visible. This is a worrying feature and is associated with poor view at laryngoscopy.

3.2.2.2 *Thyromental distance*

Measured between the tip of the thyroid cartilage and the mentum, with the neck in maximal extension, this distance should be >6.5 cm. Distances less than this are associated with poor views at laryngoscopy.

3.2.2.3 *Jaw protrusion*

The ability of the patient to protrude the lower incisors forward of the upper is assessed. Limitation of jaw protrusion (particularly if the lower teeth cannot even be brought into alignment with the upper teeth) is associated with difficulty at laryngoscopy.

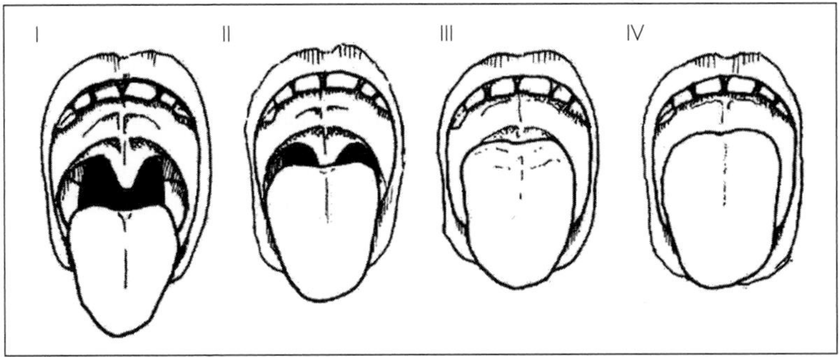

Fig 3.2 Mallampati grading.

Reproduced from Allman and Wilson, *Oxford Handbook of Anaesthesia* 3rd edition, 2011, page 972 with permission from Oxford University Press.

3.2.3 **Consent**

The final stage of the assessment is to gain the patient's consent for the anaesthetic.

The following is provided for information purposes. It is recognized that an anaesthetist in the earliest stages of their training may not be able to consent patients themselves, particularly in complex situations or those involving children. However, having some awareness of the issues is useful so that they can recognize these situations and seek advice or assistance as appropriate.

To give consent, the patient must have received adequate information to reach a judgement with which they feel comfortable. The amount of information a person requires is highly individual, and the anaesthetist should be flexible in how they communicate with different patients.

The patient must be given sufficient time to reach their decision without pressure, be able to retain the information long enough to weigh the options, and then be able to communicate their choice. They do not necessarily have to remember the conversation in the longer term, so some patients with memory impairment will still be able to offer valid consent.

Note that, under English law, no one can give consent on behalf of another adult, unless they possess a document giving them lasting power of attorney. The situation differs under Scots law.

Unexpected events occasionally occur during anaesthesia, making it necessary to perform a procedure for which the patient has not explicitly consented. It is reasonable to proceed in the patient's best interests, provided that the anaesthetist is satisfied that the patient would not object. Care must be taken for patients who have an advance directive.

With children, a person with parental responsibility can give or withhold consent. The child's mother always has this responsibility (unless it is removed by order of a court of law); however, a child's father may not always have parental responsibility. Although seldom an issue, if there is doubt with regard to the validity of consent, the advice of senior colleagues should be sought immediately. Some older children may be competent to give consent on their own behalf, even if under 16 years of age, if the doctor concerned can be satisfied that they fully understand the implications of the decision. This is not something that a junior trainee would be expected to determine.

3.2.4 **ASA grading**

The American Society of Anesthesiologists (ASA) has developed a grading system to classify patients by the severity of their comorbidities. Although somewhat vague and subjective, the system is a convenient way of communicating the complexity of a patient.

- **ASA 1:** a fit and healthy patient with no comorbidities
- **ASA 2:** a patient with mild systemic disease, such as well-controlled asthma, that does not limit their day-to-day activities
- **ASA 3:** a patient with moderate to severe systemic disease that has limiting effects. Examples might include stable angina
- **ASA 4:** a patient with severe systemic disease that is a constant threat to life. This could include unstable angina
- **ASA 5:** a moribund patient who is not expected to survive without immediate surgery. An example might include ruptured abdominal aortic aneurysm

- **ASA 6:** this grade is reserved for the brain-dead patient submitted for organ retrieval surgery
- **'E' suffix:** is appended to the ASA grade of a patient submitted for emergency surgery.

3.2.5 NCEPOD grading

The National Confidential Enquiry into Patient Outcome and Death (NCEPOD) has produced guidelines for grading operations by their urgency.

- **Immediate:** the planned intervention is immediately life- or limb-saving, and surgery should take place within minutes of the decision to operate being made
- **Urgent:** surgery is required for acute-onset conditions, or those with clinical deterioration, in a potentially life-threatening situation, or those with conditions that may threaten survival of a limb or organ. Normally, surgery is carried out within hours of the decision to proceed being made
- **Expedited:** the patient requires early treatment of a condition that is not immediately life- or limb-threatening. Intervention usually occurs within days of the decision to operate
- **Elective:** a preplanned procedure timed to suit the patient and hospital.

The same operation may fall into several categories, depending on the nature of the patient's pathology. NCEPOD gives the example of hemicolectomy, which, in the context of life-threatening GI bleeding, would require immediate surgery; however, in the case of perforated large bowel, surgery would be urgent. Large bowel obstruction would require expedited surgery, whereas a non-obstructing carcinoma could be scheduled for elective surgery.

3.3 Preoperative investigations

The National Institute for Health and Clinical Excellence (NICE) has produced a guideline with recommendations for preoperative investigations. Investigations should be targeted to answering a specific question, not ordered indiscriminately.

To decide what tests are required, the anaesthetist should consider the patient's comorbidities and the magnitude of surgery. Minor surgery includes minimally invasive, superficial operations such as incision and drainage of an abscess or excision of skin lesions. Intermediate surgery includes hernia repairs and arthroscopy. Major surgery typically involves body cavities or operations with a greater degree of physiological disturbance and could include abdominal hysterectomy or laparotomy.

Broadly, fit and well (ASA 1) patients undergoing minor surgery require no routine investigations. The only exception is the patient over 80, who should routinely have an ECG recorded. An ECG may be indicated in younger patients, but this should be determined on a case-by-case basis. Similarly, blood samples are seldom of use and should only be requested if a specific question can be addressed by the result. ASA 1 patients undergoing more significant surgery may require more detailed investigation, depending on age and the nature of the case. Fig 3.3 summarizes the current recommendations by the NICE guidelines for investigations, based on the degree of surgery.

Preoperative investigation recommendations

Adapted from NICE CG3: Preoperative Tests

Key

40 60 80 All — Recommended
This test is likely to be valuable in all patients above displayed age, and performing it would generally be recommended

40 60 80 All — Consider
This test may have value in some patients and should be considered for those above displayed age if there is a specific indication

Not recommended
This test would generally not be valuable for these patients

1. What is the patient's ASA grade?

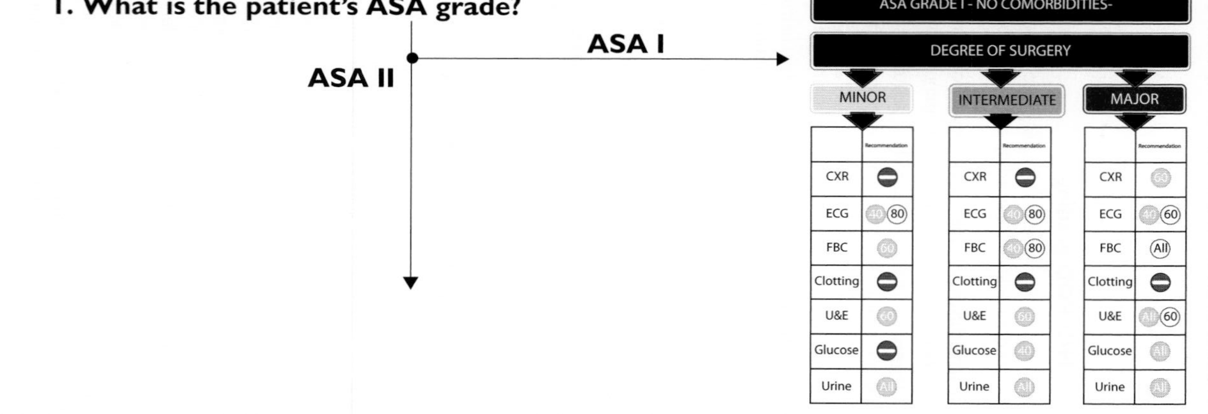

MINOR

	Recommendation
CXR	—
ECG	40 80
FBC	60
Clotting	—
U&E	60
Glucose	—
Urine	All

INTERMEDIATE

	Recommendation
CXR	—
ECG	40 80
FBC	40 80
Clotting	—
U&E	60
Glucose	40
Urine	All

MAJOR

	Recommendation
CXR	60
ECG	40 60
FBC	All
Clotting	—
U&E	All 60
Glucose	All
Urine	All

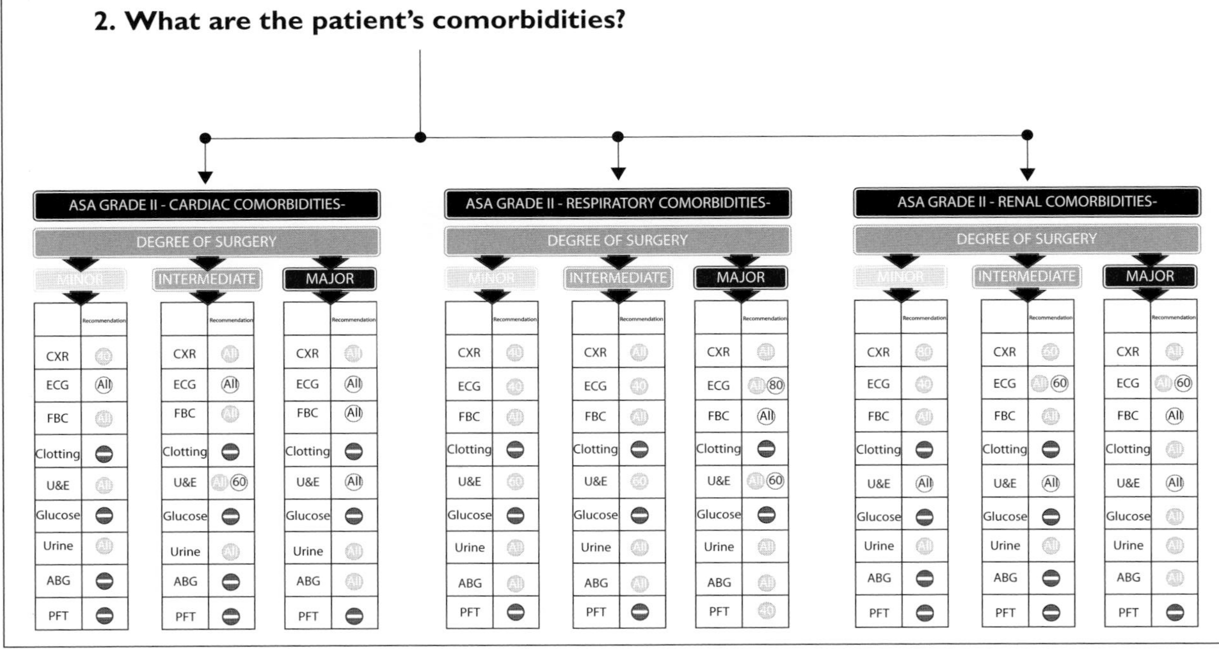

Fig 3.3 A summary of NICE guidelines *CG3: preoperative tests* (published in 2003), illustrating investigations indicated for ASA 1 and 2 patients undergoing varying degrees of surgery.

Patients with mild systemic disease (ASA 2) can benefit from routine investigations, depending on the nature of their illness and the degree of surgery.

This chapter focuses on ASA 1 and 2 adult patients undergoing minor or intermediate surgery, as these are of most relevance to the new anaesthetist. It should be noted that patients with more complex needs, or those undergoing more significant surgery, require a more detailed investigation.

3.3.1 **Cardiovascular disease**

All patients with cardiovascular disease should have an ECG preoperatively. Other investigations, such as blood tests, may be indicated for certain patients, e.g biochemistry for all patients taking diuretic therapy or patients aged over 60 undergoing intermediate surgery.

3.3.2 **Respiratory disease**

Patients with mild disease, such as well-controlled asthma, may require no investigations. Consideration can be given to other investigations on a case-by-case basis, but invasive tests, such as blood gas sampling, or radiography are seldom indicated for minor or intermediate surgery.

3.3.3 **Renal disease**

All patients with renal disease should have their biochemistry checked. Other investigations, such as full blood count testing or ECG recording, can be helpful in some patients but would not be automatically required for minor surgery. An ECG would, however, be routinely requested for the older renal patient requiring intermediate surgery.

3.3.4 **Sickle-cell tests**

All patients from North or West African, South or sub-Saharan African, or Afro-Caribbean backgrounds should be asked if they are aware of their sickle-cell status. If their status is unknown, testing for sickle-cell anaemia would be recommended, particularly if there is a family history of the condition.

Note that the sickle-gene is also present in communities from Eastern Mediterranean, the Middle East, and Asia.

3.3.5 **Pregnancy testing**

Female patients of reproductive age should be asked if there is a possibility of pregnancy. Any patient who feels there is a possibility of pregnancy, or has an uncertain menstrual history, should be formally tested where either the surgery or the anaesthetic technique could have adverse effects on a fetus.

3.3.6 **Consent**

The standard principles of informed consent apply to preoperative investigations, and patients should be informed of the indication for testing, particularly if a positive result would have long-term consequences for the patient. This is particularly important for pregnancy tests or sickle-cell tests.

3.4 Planning a general anaesthetic

Safe anaesthesia requires the assimilation of a number of sources of data and the synthesis of a plan. The anaesthetic can be loosely broken down into three stages to aid preparation: induction, maintenance, and emergence. At each of the steps, a number of choices need to be made about appropriate techniques or medications. Some of these are illustrated in Fig 3.4.

It can seem quite complicated, but a checklist (see Fig 3.5) can help the anaesthetist to remember each of the components of the process that need to be considered.

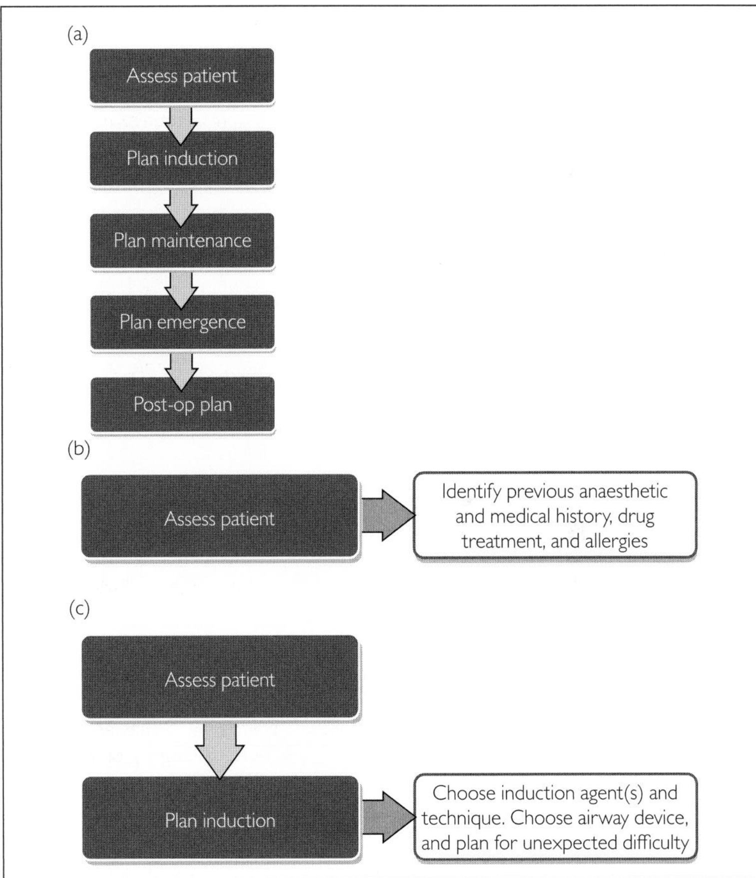

Fig 3.4 This flow chart illustrates the various steps of a general anaesthetic and the issues which should be considered at each point (see a–j). A video of this is available in the video appendix. Once the user hits play, the video will automatically show each sequence.

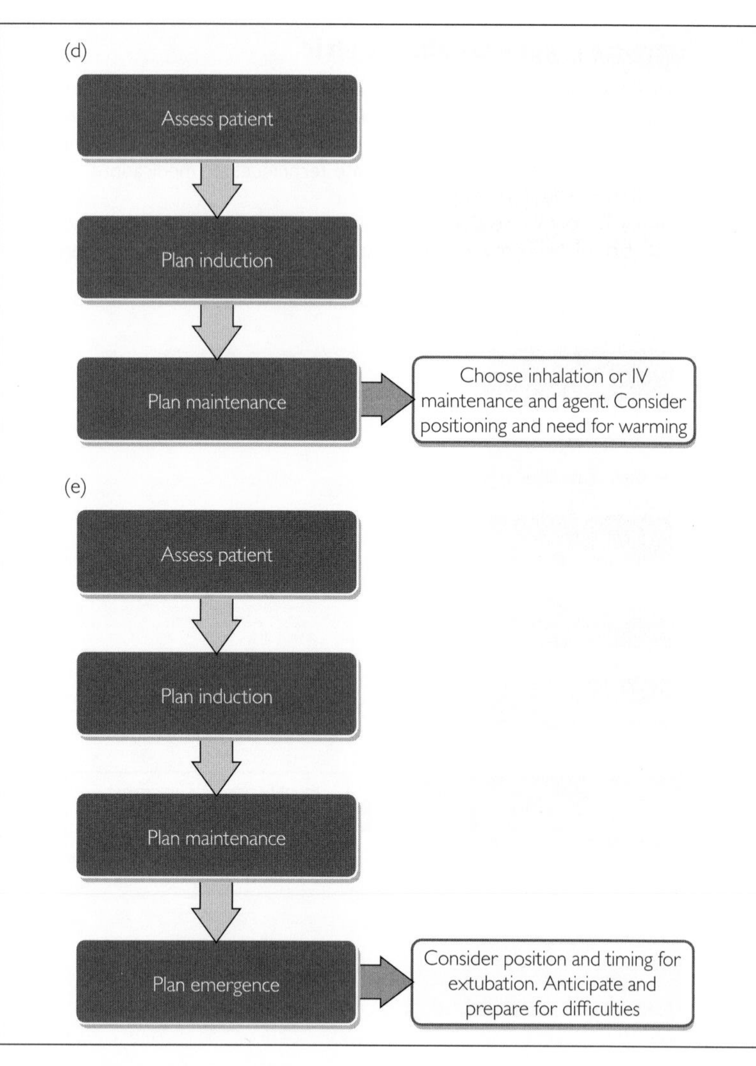
(d)
Assess patient
Plan induction
Plan maintenance
Choose inhalation or IV maintenance and agent. Consider positioning and need for warming
(e)
Assess patient
Plan induction
Plan maintenance
Plan emergence
Consider position and timing for extubation. Anticipate and prepare for difficulties

Fig 3.4 Continued

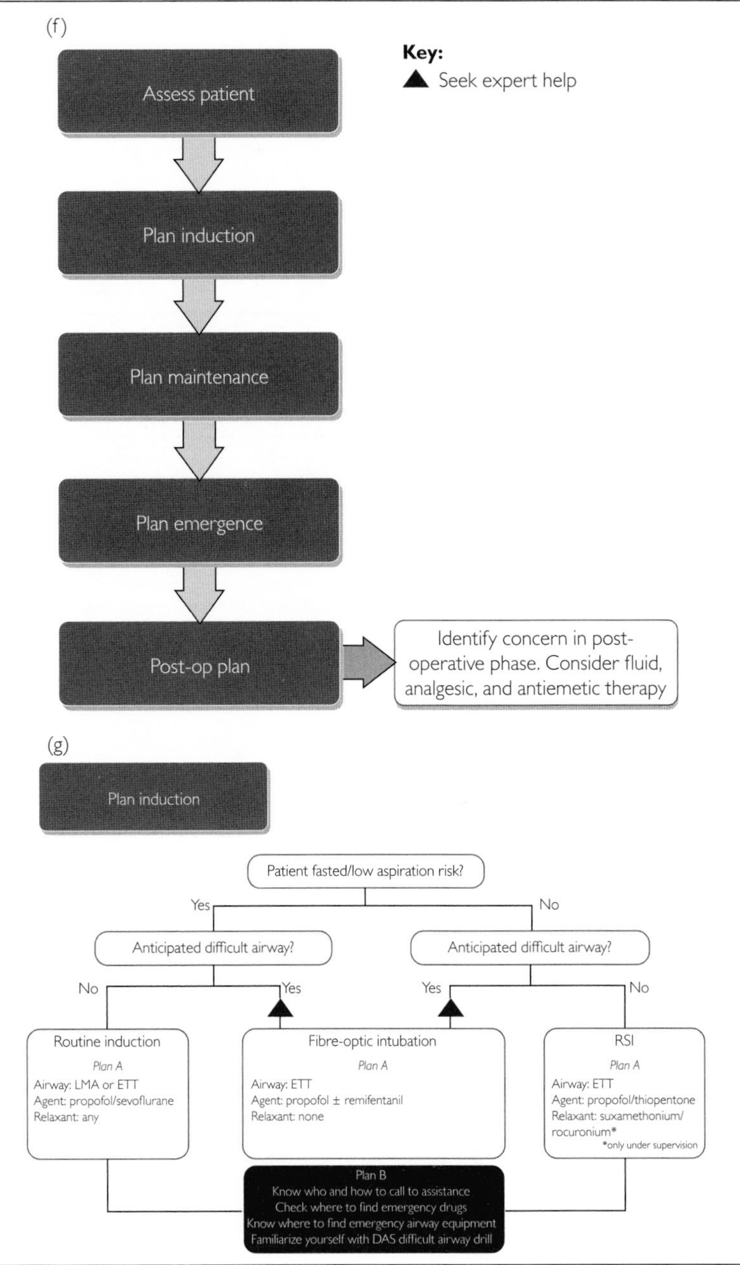
(f)
Key:
Seek expert help
Assess patient
Plan induction
Plan maintenance
Plan emergence
Post-op plan
Identify concern in post-operative phase. Consider fluid, analgesic, and antiemetic therapy
(g)
Plan induction
Patient fasted/low aspiration risk?
Yes
No
Anticipated difficult airway?
Anticipated difficult airway?
No
Yes
Yes
No
Routine induction
Plan A
Airway: LMA or ETT
Agent: propofol/sevoflurane
Relaxant: any
Fibre-optic intubation
Plan A
Airway: ETT
Agent: propofol ± remifentanil
Relaxant: none
RSI
Plan A
Airway: ETT
Agent: propofol/thiopentone
Relaxant: suxamethonium/rocuronium*
*only under supervision
Plan B
Know who and how to call to assistance
Check where to find emergency drugs
Know where to find emergency airway equipment
Familiarize yourself with DAS difficult airway drill

Fig 3.4 Continued

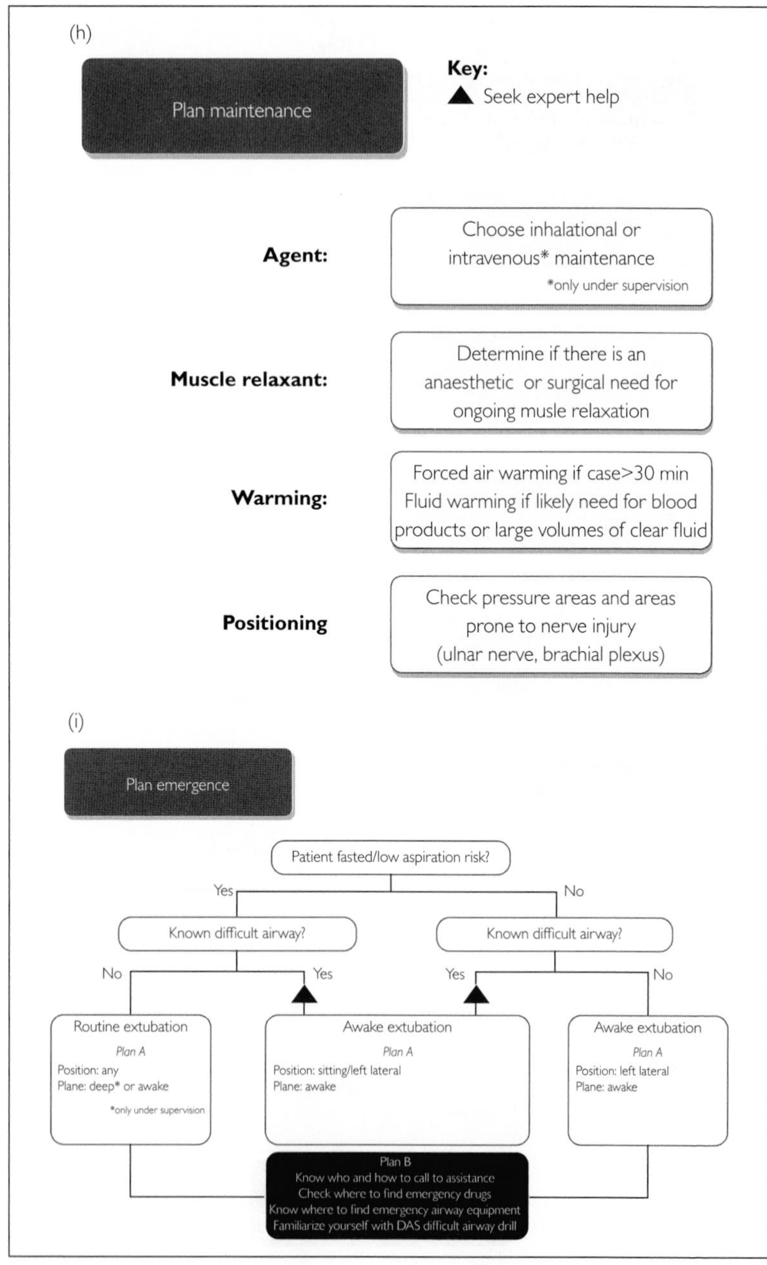

(h)
Plan maintenance
Key:
▲ Seek expert help
Agent:
Choose inhalational or intravenous* maintenance
*only under supervision
Muscle relaxant:
Determine if there is an anaesthetic or surgical need for ongoing musle relaxation
Warming:
Forced air warming if case>30 min
Fluid warming if likely need for blood products or large volumes of clear fluid
Positioning
Check pressure areas and areas prone to nerve injury
(ulnar nerve, brachial plexus)
(i)
Plan emergence
Patient fasted/low aspiration risk?
Yes
No
Known difficult airway?
Known difficult airway?
No
Yes
Yes
No
Routine extubation
Plan A
Position: any
Plane: deep* or awake
*only under supervision
Awake extubation
Plan A
Position: sitting/left lateral
Plane: awake
Awake extubation
Plan A
Position: left lateral
Plane: awake
Plan B
Know who and how to call to assistance
Check where to find emergency drugs
Know where to find emergency airway equipment
Familiarize yourself with DAS difficult airway drill

Fig 3.4 Continued

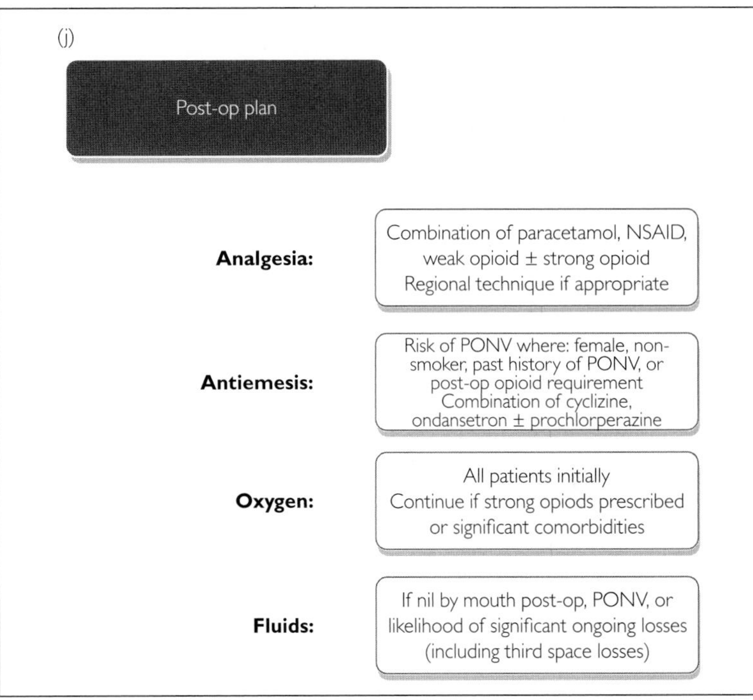

(j)
Post-op plan
Analgesia:
Combination of paracetamol, NSAID, weak opioid ± strong opioid
Regional technique if appropriate
Antiemesis:
Risk of PONV where: female, non-smoker, past history of PONV, or post-op opioid requirement
Combination of cyclizine, ondansetron ± prochlorperazine
Oxygen:
All patients initially
Continue if strong opiods prescribed or significant comorbidities
Fluids:
If nil by mouth post-op, PONV, or likelihood of significant ongoing losses (including third space losses)

Fig 3.4 Continued

3.4.1 **Induction**

Induction is one of the periods associated with highest risk during anaesthesia. Most problems are either airway-related or cardiovascular (in particular, hypotension); however, the majority of these problems are predictable and can be managed with appropriate planning.

3.4.1.1 *Venue*

The anaesthetist must choose first where the induction will take place. In the UK, most anaesthetics begin in the anaesthetic room, but a proportion of patients might be better anaesthetized in theatre. Patients in need of immediate surgery (e.g. life-threatening bleeding) are often anaesthetized on the operating table to minimize delay between induction and start of surgery. Similarly, the morbidly obese patient may be anaesthetized in theatre to minimize transfers and manual handling risks. In such cases, a senior anaesthetist should be present to assist.

3.4.1.2 *Airway*

The anaesthetist must choose the most appropriate airway device for the case. In the patient at risk of aspiration (e.g. emergency surgery in the non-fasted patient), a tracheal tube is almost always indicated.

Anaesthetic planning checklist

Operation	
Venue for induction	
Airway device	
Ventilation mode	
Induction agent	
Muscle relaxant	
Maintenance agent	
Emergence plan	
Analgesia	
Post-operative care	

Fig 3.5 An example of a checklist that could be used to help planning a general anaesthetic.

A tracheal tube would also often be required for patients undergoing surgery that involves the airway (many ENT or Max-Fax operations) and operations that require muscle relaxation to facilitate surgery. A range of different tube types is available, depending on the specifics of the case.

Short cases in fasted patients that do not present an airway risk are most commonly conducted using a laryngeal mask.

3.4.1.3 *Breathing*

The choice between spontaneous and mechanical ventilation must also be made.

Any patient requiring muscle relaxation (see Section 2.4) must be mechanically ventilated for the duration of the neuromuscular blockade.

Most patients will be apnoeic for a period after induction, so almost all patients will require some manual or mechanical ventilation at induction.

At induction, the patient should receive 100% oxygen (fractional inspired oxygen concentration, or F_iO_2, of 1.0) whilst still awake, and this should continue until the airway has been secured.

3.4.1.4 *Circulation*

Induction agents can cause significant hypotension, so a plan to manage this, particularly where a significant fall in blood pressure can be predicted (e.g. the patient with pre-existing hypertension or the hypovolaemic patient), is necessary. The anaesthetist should decide what limits for hypotension are acceptable. Drops in mean arterial pressure (MAP) of up to 25% during anaesthesia are usually acceptable without adverse consequences, but consider treating falls larger than this. In patients with cardiac or cerebrovascular disease, it may be more appropriate to maintain MAP at, or close to, pre-induction values.

Most patients require IV fluids for all but short-duration cases, particularly where significant blood loss is expected. Fluids should be warmed if volumes above 2 L are likely to be used, or where blood products will be transfused.

The anaesthetist should prepare vasopressors (typically metaraminol or phenylephrine) and/or inotropes (usually ephedrine) before a case where the patient would be put at risk by a period of hypotension or where larger drops in MAP are predicted (see Section 2.5.1).

Plans should be made to deal with arrhythmias in the at-risk patient. Wherever possible, their medical management must be optimized before surgery, and the anaesthetist may require additional drugs (e.g. digoxin, amiodarone) or equipment (defibrillator or pacemaker) to be available.

3.4.1.5 *Drugs*

The choice of IV (see Section 2.2) or inhalational induction (see Section 2.3.1) should be made. IV induction is the most common method in adult practice.

Propofol is often considered the 'default' IV agent, as it has useful properties in terms of suppression of airway reflexes and antiemesis, but sodium thiopental is useful for RSI, as it has a more predictable dose–response than propofol and is non-irritant on IV injection.

Inhalational inductions using sevoflurane are commonly performed in children and under certain circumstances in adults. An inhalational induction for those patients who will not or cannot have IV access secured beforehand is a riskier technique. If the patient develops laryngospasm before IV access has been secured, it is much more difficult to treat. Inhalational inductions for such patients should only be conducted with the assistance of an experienced anaesthetist.

A choice of muscle relaxant drugs is available. Suxamethonium (see Section 2.4.2.1) is usually reserved for RSI (see Section 5.2) and emergency management of laryngospasm (see Section 7.5.3). After a dose of suxamethonium, if ongoing muscle relaxation is required, a longer-acting drug will also be required (see Section 2.4.1).

Drugs, such as atracurium, rocuronium, or vecuronium, are suitable for muscle relaxation in routine inductions and for maintenance of muscle relaxation after an RSI.

3.4.1.6 *Everything else*

All patients should be optimized as far as possible before coming to theatre. This means ensuring, at a minimum, that their medical conditions are adequately controlled and that they are volume-replete. Any outstanding results of investigations should be available.

3.4.2 **Maintenance**

After a single dose of propofol or thiopental the patient would be expected to wake in 5–10 min, so maintenance phase begins after the airway has been secured and drugs to continue general anaesthesia have been introduced.

There are some important decisions that should be made with regard to maintenance of anaesthesia.

3.4.2.1 *Airway*

This will have been determined by the choice of airway selected on induction. In very few cases would a change of airway be planned.

3.4.2.2 *Breathing*

All patients will require an oxygen-enriched gas supply (usually F_iO_2 >0.3) during maintenance, as all anaesthetic agents worsen the V/Q mismatch. Prolonged exposure to high oxygen concentrations can be harmful, so a second gas is introduced to reduce the F_iO_2. Usually, this second gas is medical air, but nitrous oxide (see Section 2.3.4) may have advantages in some patients.

The rationale for deciding maintenance ventilation mode is similar to that made at induction. Mechanical ventilation is mandatory if neuromuscular blockers have been given. Patients requiring prolonged operations may also benefit from mechanical ventilation (see Section 1.2.10).

The choice between mechanical and spontaneous respiration does not necessarily depend on the choice of airway. It is common to mechanically ventilate patients using an LMA, and it is possible to self-ventilate on a tracheal tube after the muscle relaxant has fully worn off.

It may be appropriate to allow spontaneous respiration in some phases of the case and mechanical ventilation during others.

3.4.2.3 *Circulation*

Much as at induction, the anaesthetist must have a trigger at which hypotension should be treated. The anaesthetist should also determine what volume of IV fluids might be required and at what rate they should be administered. These decisions will be informed by the preoperative volume state, ongoing losses (bleeding and insensible), and cardiovascular measurements such as heart rate and blood pressure.

Tachycardia or hypertension can usually be treated by deepening anaesthesia or by administering analgesics (most often a rapidly acting opioid such as fentanyl— see Section 2.6.3).

3.4.2.4 *Drugs*

Under most circumstances, anaesthesia is maintained using an inhalational agent— sevoflurane, isoflurane, or desflurane (see Section 2.3).

Sevoflurane is useful as an induction agent, as it has rapid onset/offset and is pleasant to breathe, but its advantages over isoflurane as a maintenance agent are less clear. It is also more expensive.

The unique physical properties of desflurane mean that it can be more difficult to use; some hospitals reserve it for use by more experienced anaesthetists. Similarly, TIVA techniques with propofol and remifentanil require more experience to use safely, not least because it is harder to assess the depth of anaesthesia because the concentration of the drug cannot be monitored. There is no MAC equivalent for a TIVA technique. TIVA is also more difficult to use when an RSI is required.

Depth of anaesthesia is most easily determined during inhalational maintenance, as the end-tidal agent concentration can be measured. Patients should be maintained at values >1 MAC to reduce the risk of awareness.

The analgesic plan is usually started at some point during the maintenance phase, initially with short-acting opioids, such as fentanyl, and with non-opioid analgesics like paracetamol or diclofenac. Towards the end of a case, it may be appropriate to start giving longer-acting opioids such as morphine.

3.4.2.5 *Everything else*

Patients under general anaesthesia vasodilate; combined with the administration of cold fluids and gases, hypothermia is common. The heat and moisture exchange (HME) filter included in the breathing circuit goes some way to warming and humidifying airway gases, but consideration should be given to actively warming all patients undergoing surgery longer than 30 min. This is achieved with a forced-air warming device that blows warmed air through a specialized blanket. Fluid warming is appropriate for longer, more complex cases.

3.4.3 **Emergence**

Like induction, emergence is associated with significant risks, usually related to airway management. Good planning and preparation can help to minimize these risks.

3.4.3.1 *Airway*

Patients with a laryngeal mask in place who are otherwise stable and self-ventilating can be taken to recovery with the LMA in place. Patients with a tracheal tube need to be extubated and stabilized before leaving theatre.

The Difficult Airway Society (DAS) has produced guidelines to help planning for extubation (see Figs 3.6a–c). The key decision is between deep and awake extubation; the majority of extubations are conducted awake, and deep extubation should only be performed under supervision (see Section 7.5).

The tube should not be removed if there is any doubt that it can be promptly replaced in the event of problems, and the patient should be otherwise stable, fully preoxygenated, and responding to voice before the tube is removed. Further details can be found in the chapter dealing with airway problems at extubation.

3.4.3.2 *Breathing*

Neuromuscular blockade must be fully reversed before the patient is woken up.

All patients must be properly preoxygenated prior to emergence and continue on high-flow oxygen until fully awake. All patients should be self-ventilating prior to leaving theatre.

3.4.3.3 *Circulation*

Most patients will become tachycardic, with or without hypertension, as anaesthesia lightens. This seldom requires intervention, but a small proportion of patients may be at risk from the increased cardiac oxygen demands.

3.4.3.4 *Drugs*

The most important drugs prior to emergence are analgesics to ensure patient comfort on waking and reversal of neuromuscular blockade. If a muscle relaxant has been used,

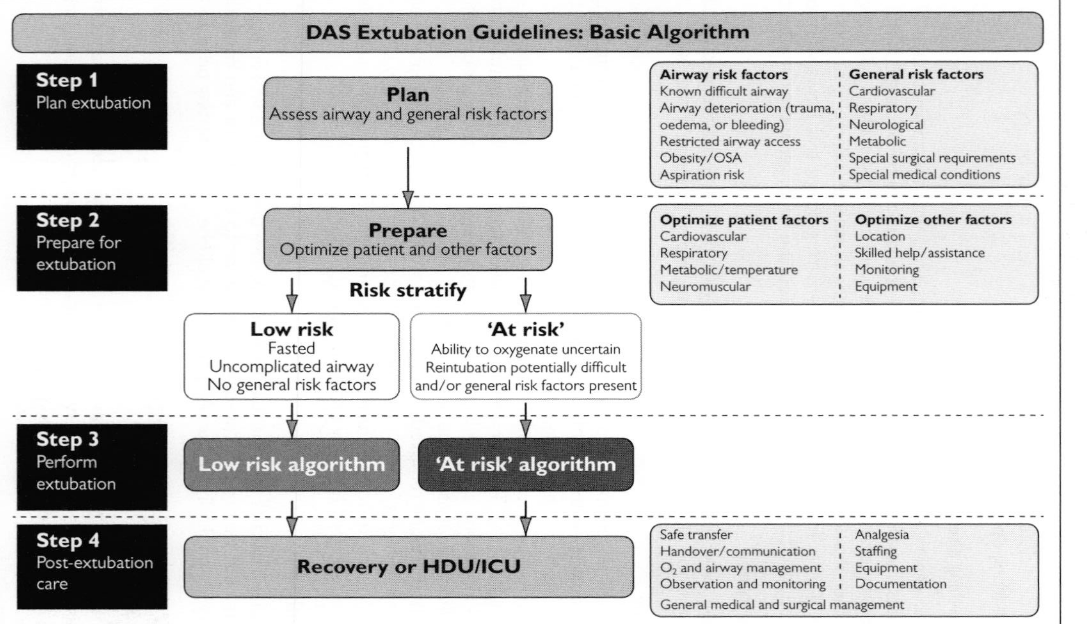

Fig 3.6a Guidelines produced by the Difficult Airway Society (2011) to help planning for extubation.

Reproduced with permission from the Difficult Airway Society.

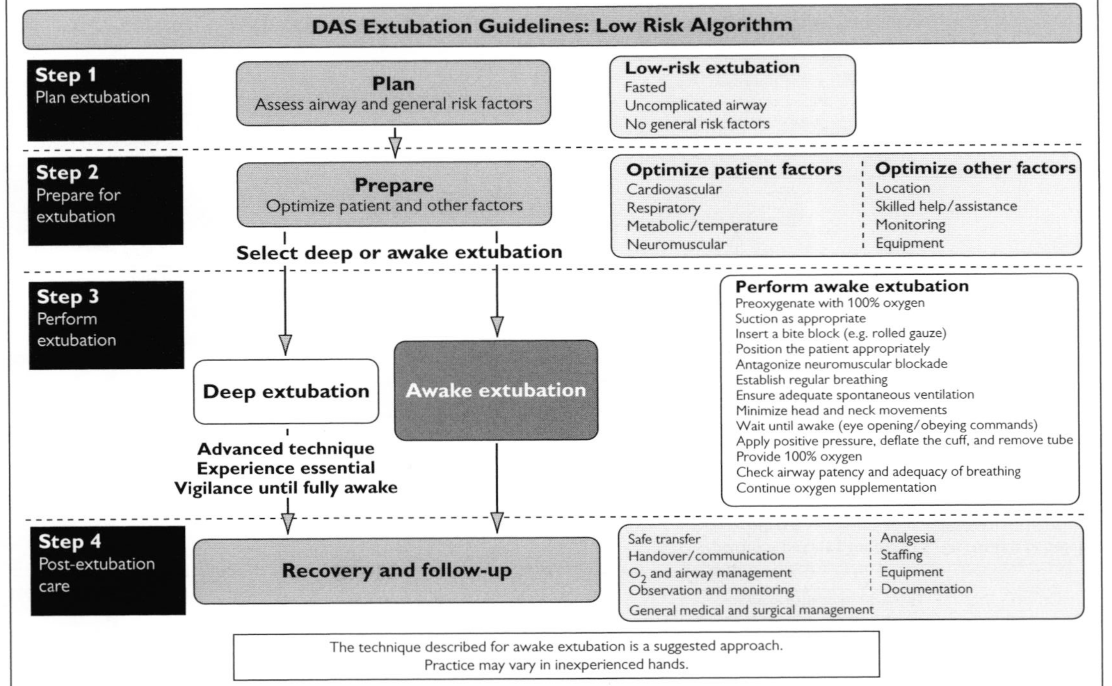

Fig 3.6b Guidelines produced by the Difficult Airway Society (2011) to help planning for the extubation of a low-risk airway.
Reproduced with permission from the Difficult Airway Society.

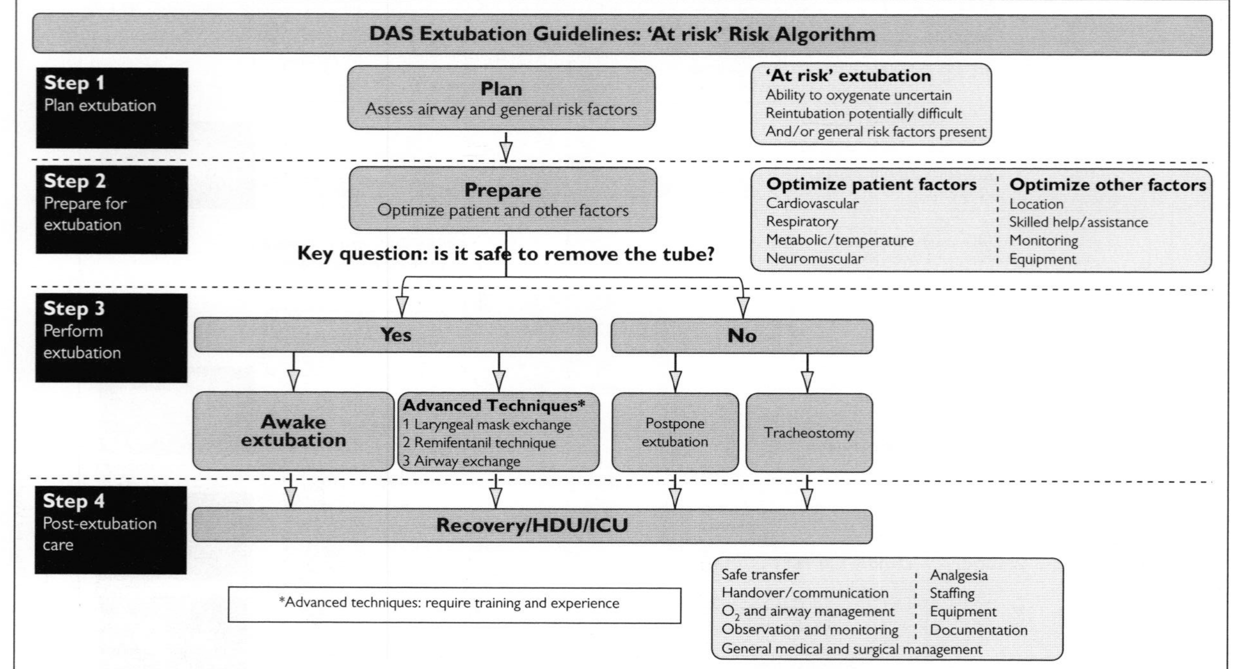

Fig 3.6c Guidelines produced by the Difficult Airway Society (2011) to help planning for the extubation of a high-risk airway.

it is mandatory to assess the level of residual block with a nerve stimulator prior to emergence and then to administer neostigmine and glycopyrrolate, if indicated (see Section 2.4.3.1).

3.4.3.5 *Everything else*

The anaesthetist should plan how to access help in the event of a problem and mentally prepare their sequence of actions in the event of problems such as laryngospasm (see Section 7.5.3).

3.4.4 **Post-operative care**

Before the patient leaves theatre, a plan for their analgesic and fluid therapy should be documented.

Analgesics (see Section 2.6) are usually prescribed according to the WHO analgesic ladder (see Fig 3.7), starting with paracetamol and adding an NSAID as required. These are usually best prescribed on a regular basis. Next steps include weak opioids, then strong opioids, often on an 'as-required' basis.

All patients should have oxygen prescribed. Antiemesis (see Section 2.7) and IV fluids should be considered.

If there have been unexpected difficulties during the case, some consideration should be given to whether a period of high dependency or intensive care might be appropriate.

3.4.5 **Example case plans**

3.4.5.1 *Elective knee arthroscopy*

See Fig 3.8.

History: a 28-year-old male, with no past medical history of note, is attending for an elective day-case right knee arthroscopy. Previous general anaesthetics have been

WHO analgesic ladder

Minimal pain	Mild pain	Moderate pain	Severe pain	
			Morphine 15–30 mg[PO] 2-hourly	Strong opioid
		Codeine 30–60 mg 4–6-hourly	Codeine 30–60 mg 4–6-hourly	Weak opioid
	Ibuprofen 400 mg 4–6-hourly	Ibuprofen 400 mg 4–6-hourly	Ibuprofen 400 mg 4–6-hourly	NSAID
Paracetamol 1 g 4–6-hourly	Paracetamol 1 g 4–6-hourly	Paracetamol 1 g 4–6-hourly	Paracetamol 1 g 4–6-hourly	Simple analgesia

Avoid NSAIDs where:
Allergy to NSAIDs
Coagulopathy
NSAID-sensitive asthma
Renal impairment
Caution at extremes of age

Fig 3.7 An illustration of the WHO analgesic ladder.
Reproduced with permission from the World Health Organization <http://www.who.int/cancer/palliative/painladder/en/>.

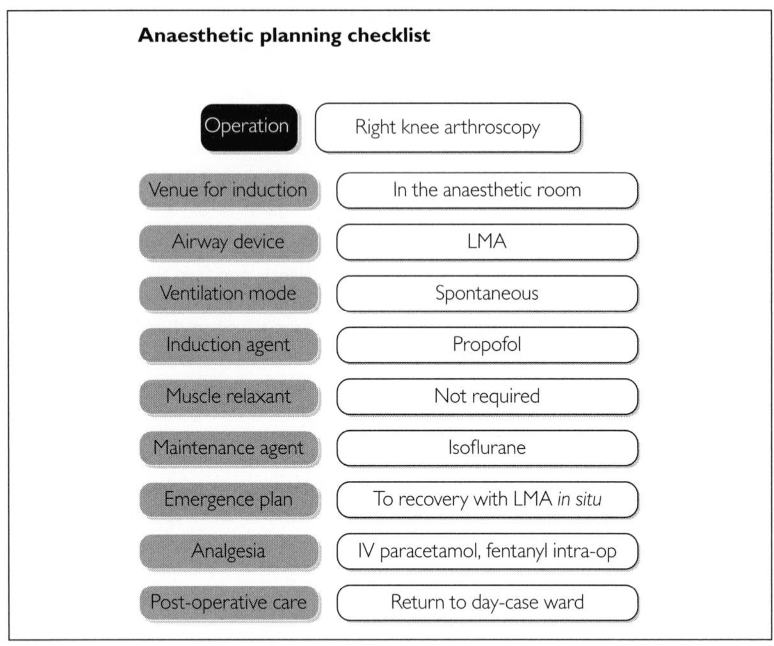

Anaesthetic planning checklist
Operation
Right knee arthroscopy
Venue for induction
In the anaesthetic room
Airway device
LMA
Ventilation mode
Spontaneous
Induction agent
Propofol
Muscle relaxant
Not required
Maintenance agent
Isoflurane
Emergence plan
To recovery with LMA in situ
Analgesia
IV paracetamol, fentanyl intra-op
Post-operative care
Return to day-case ward

Fig 3.8 An example checklist that has been completed for a patient undergoing a knee arthroscopy.

unremarkable, and he has no allergies. The patient is fasted, and the airway assessment is reassuring.

Plan: the case can safely be induced in the anaesthetic room, and, as he is fasted, an LMA is appropriate. Muscle relaxation is not required to assist surgery, so he can spontaneously ventilate. Anaesthesia can be induced with propofol and maintained with isoflurane. If there are no unexpected events, he can wake in recovery with the LMA *in situ* and return to the day-case ward when alert. Analgesia can be achieved using IV paracetamol and IV fentanyl in theatre, and regular ibuprofen post-operatively combined with PRN codeine. 'Rescue' fentanyl should be prescribed for use in the recovery room. The patient should be safe to discharge home 3–4 h post-operatively if he remains well.

3.4.5.2 *Urgent laparoscopic appendicectomy*

See Fig 3.9.

History: a 36-year-old female presents with a 3-day history of worsening right iliac fossa pain, increased inflammatory markers, and ultrasound features consistent with appendicitis. She has a past history of asthma, for which she takes inhaled salbutamol as required and twice-daily beclomethasone. Her asthma has been well controlled recently; she has never had oral steroids or been admitted with acute severe asthma.

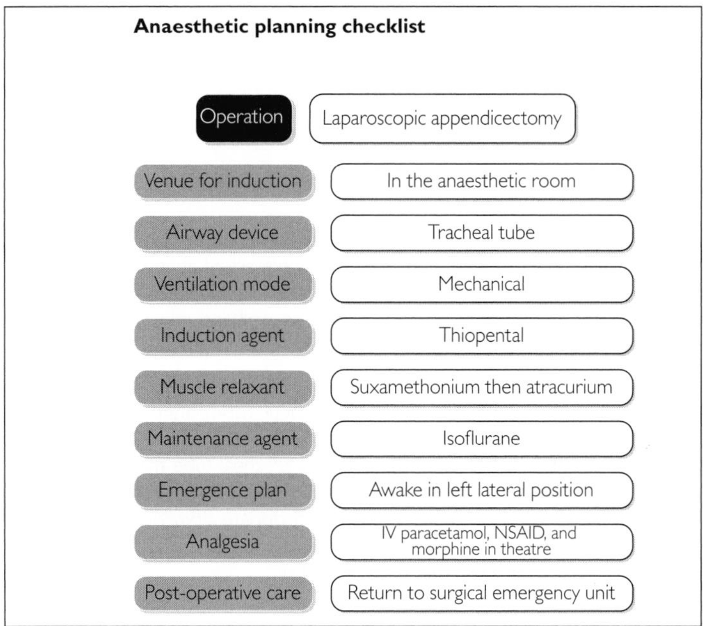

Anaesthetic planning checklist
Operation
Laparoscopic appendicectomy
Venue for induction
In the anaesthetic room
Airway device
Tracheal tube
Ventilation mode
Mechanical
Induction agent
Thiopental
Muscle relaxant
Suxamethonium then atracurium
Maintenance agent
Isoflurane
Emergence plan
Awake in left lateral position
Analgesia
IV paracetamol, NSAID, and morphine in theatre
Post-operative care
Return to surgical emergency unit

Fig 3.9 An example checklist that has been completed for a patient undergoing a laparoscopic appendicectomy.

She tolerates NSAIDs without any problems. She is allergic to penicillin, which causes a rash. Her airway assessment is unremarkable, and she is fasted. She is certain that she is not pregnant.

Plan: this patient is unwell, but stable, so can safely be anaesthetized in the anaesthetic room. Even though she has not eaten for >6 h, in the context of an acute abdomen, gastric emptying cannot be relied upon, so an RSI technique is indicated. Classically this would use sodium thiopental with suxamethonium. Laparoscopy requires pneumoperitoneum, which raises intra-abdominal pressures. Since this would make spontaneous ventilation difficult, mechanical ventilation is indicated. Continued muscle relaxation may also assist the surgeons. Atracurium would be an appropriate choice after the suxamethonium had worn off.

Isoflurane would be appropriate as a maintenance agent. Fentanyl may be given shortly before the first incision, and, as pain can be a feature post-operatively, a strong opioid such as morphine, in combination with IV paracetamol, would be beneficial prior to awakening.

After a rapid sequence technique, awake extubation is usually mandatory and is generally conducted in the left lateral position to reduce the risk of airway soiling. The tube should only be removed with the patient opening eyes to voice or making purposeful movements.

After a short period in recovery, the patient should be able to go to the surgical emergency unit for ongoing care. Post-operative analgesia on the ward will probably include paracetamol, ibuprofen, codeine, and oral morphine. The use of long-acting opioids means that oxygen should be prescribed and she will probably need IV fluid maintenance until her oral intake normalizes.

3.4.5.3 *Dental extractions*

See Fig 3.10.

History: a 29-year-old male presents for elective extraction of all four '8s'. This will be his first anaesthetic, although there is no family history of anaesthetic problems. He is a smoker and has previously had difficulties with alcohol misuse, although he has not drunk alcohol for several months. He is otherwise well and takes no regular medications. He has no allergies.

His dental condition is poor, but his airway assessment is reassuring. He is fasted.

Plan: he can safely be anaesthetized in the anaesthetic room, although some dental lists anaesthetize their patients on the operating table to reduce the time taken for each case.

As this surgery requires access to the airway, a tracheal tube may be indicated. It is possible to conduct simple extractions under an LMA, and this should be discussed with the operating surgeon to determine the most appropriate airway choice.

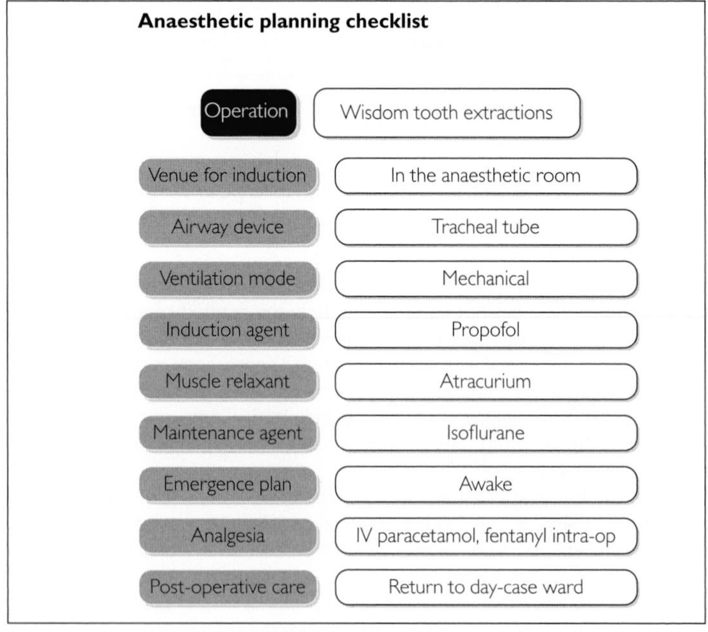

Fig 3.10 An example checklist that has been completed for a patient undergoing wisdom tooth extraction.

As he is fasted he does not require an RSI and propofol would be appropriate, along with atracurium if intubation is performed. Muscle relaxation would mandate mechanical ventilation.

Anaesthesia can be maintained with isoflurane. The potential for blood in the airway means that an awake extubation at the end of the case would be most appropriate. The surgeon will inject LA, so pain should be manageable with a combination of paracetamol and fentanyl. Rescue analgesia, with either fentanyl or morphine, should be prescribed for recovery.

Assuming no complications, he can be safely discharged from recovery to the day-case unit, with a combination of paracetamol, ibuprofen, and codeine.

3.5 Communication in theatre

A large team of people is required to make a theatre function effectively, and the patient undergoing even minor surgery could easily have contact with >20 people during their admission. No person functions in isolation, and the actions of one individual impact on the decisions and actions of others. It is therefore vital that team members communicate effectively.

Once the anaesthetic plan has been formulated, it should be discussed with the anaesthetic assistant and the surgical staff. This will ensure that appropriate drugs and equipment are available and that no elements of the anaesthetic plan conflict with the surgical plan and vice versa.

Communication in theatre is a vital 'non-technical' skill.

3.5.1 The WHO checklist

The WHO published a surgical safety checklist in 2008, which has been developed with a view to global implementation to reduce the number of complications that occur during elective and emergency surgery. The checklist has been widely adopted throughout the UK, and most theatres have preprepared stationery to aid its use (see Fig 3.11).

Surgical and anaesthetic staff are expected to meet before the first patient on the list arrives in theatre to introduce themselves by name and role. At this briefing, the general conduct of the list is discussed, including any changes to the proposed order, any expected difficulties, equipment needs, and a brief overview of surgical and anaesthetic plans. This is an ideal opportunity to discuss specific needs, such as positioning or airway choice, with the operating surgeons.

A checklist is completed for every patient as they arrive in theatre. This identifies three stages in the surgical journey and highlights a series of checks that must be completed at each step. Except under highly unusual circumstances, anaesthesia or surgery should not continue until these checks have been satisfactorily completed.

Step 1: Sign in

This is usually conducted by the anaesthetic assistant in the anaesthetic room and consists of confirmation of the patient's identity, operation, surgical site, consent, allergies, and fasting state. The patient should not be given any sedative drugs prior to the completion of these checks, although it is acceptable to establish IV access and monitoring.

After the checks are completed, the patient can be anaesthetized.

WHO surgical safety checklist

Generic checklist

SIGN IN (to be read out loud)

(Shaded questions may be asked for all patients at a prelist meeting)

Have all team members introduced themselves by name and role?

Confirm the order of the list. Is the team aware of any changes?

ANTICIPATED CRITICAL EVENTS

Surgeon reviews:
- How much blood is anticipated?
- Are there any critical or unexpected steps?
- Is all the necessary equipment for this procedure available?
- Are any special investigations required?
- If required, is an ITU bed available?

Anaesthesia team reviews:
- Are there any patient-specific concerns?
- What monitoring equipment and other specific levels of support are required, e.g. blood?
- If the patient has a difficult airway/aspiration risk, is equipment/assistance available?
- If there is a risk of blood loss >500 mL, (7 mL/kg in children), is adequate IV access/fluids available?

ANAESTHETIC ROOM—PATIENT PRESENT
- Has the patient confirmed his/her identity, site, procedure, and consent?
- Is the surgical site marked? Does this match the consent form and operation list?
- Is the anaesthesia and medical safety check completed?
- Does the patient have a known allergy?
- What is the patient's ASA grade?

Registered practitioner confirms that list has been read out.

Name:

Signature of registered practitioner

TIME OUT (to be read aloud)

Before skin incision

Have all team members introduced themselves by name and role?
(If not undertaken at prelist meeting)

Surgeon, anaesthetist, and other registered practitioners verbally confirm:
- What is the patient's name?
- What procedure, site, and position are planned?
- Have the risks due to patient positioning been discussed and any relevant positioning guidelines followed?
- Has the surgeon checked the consent form?
- Does the patient have any allergies?

Has the surgical site infection bundle been undertaken:
- Antibiotic prophylaxis been given in last 60 minutes?
- Patient warming?
- Hair removal (if applicable)?
- Glycaemic control?

Has VTE prophylaxis been undertaken?
- Yes/not applicable

Is essential imaging displayed?
- Yes/not applicable

Are there any other procedure-specific concerns or requirements?

Registered practitioner confirms that list has been read out.

Name:

Signature of registered practitioner

SIGN OUT (to be read aloud)

Before the surgeon leaves theatre

Registered practitioner verbally confirms with the team:
- Has the name of the procedure been recorded?
- Has the integrity of all instruments been checked?
- Has it been confirmed that swabs and sharps counts are complete?
- Have the specimens been labelled (including patient name)?
- Have any equipment problems been identified that need to be addressed?
- What are the key concerns for recovery and management of this patient?
- Have these been documented?

Registered practitioner confirms that list has been read out.

Name:

Signature of registered practitioner

PATIENT DETAILS

Procedure:

Date:

PATIENT ID LABEL

OMI ref: 4072

Fig 3.11 An example of a WHO surgical safety checklist.

Reproduced with permission from Oxford University Hospitals NHS Trust, adapted from *WHO Surgical Safety Checklist*, copyright 2008 with permission from the World Health Organization <http://www.who.int/patientsafety/safesurgery/ss_checklist/en/>.

Step 2: Time out

After transferring onto the operating table in theatre, a time out is held. A member of the scrub team, assisted by the surgeon, often conducts this. The time out should only be taken once the anaesthetist has established monitoring, ventilation, and maintenance of anaesthesia and can devote their attention to the process.

A verbal check of the patient's identity bracelet is conducted, and confirmation of the procedure, site, and positioning is made. The scrub staff and surgeon check the consent form.

Any new staff that were not present at the prelist briefing should identify themselves by name and role.

Predictable difficulties or critical steps should be highlighted, and the need for patient warming, antibiotic prophylaxis, and deep vein thrombosis (DVT) prophylaxis is discussed.

Once these checks are complete, surgery may begin.

Step 3: Sign out

The sign out occurs after surgery has been completed, but before both patient and surgeon leave theatre. The scrub team usually conducts it, but it should be timed so that it occurs when the anaesthetist is not occupied with patient tasks.

The check consists of a confirmation that swab, needle, and instrument counts are correct, and concerns for recovery are discussed.

3.5.2 **The anaesthetic assistant**

Anaesthetic assistants can be either trained nurses or operating department practitioners (ODP). Their role is to provide assistance to the anaesthetist at each stage of the anaesthetic process, and they should not be assigned to assist the surgical team, except under highly unusual circumstances.

The anaesthetic should not begin until the assistant is present and properly prepared. Anaesthetists differ slightly in their practice and preferences, so it is important to brief the assistant properly as to the equipment you will need and techniques you intend to perform.

It is important to manage the resource represented by the assistant carefully; it is easy, particularly during emergency situations, to overload the assistant with tasks. The anaesthetist should be mindful about prioritizing the requests made of the assistant and to recognize if their workload requires additional help.

3.5.3 **Communicating with the surgical team**

The anaesthetic and surgical teams do not work in isolation from each other. As highlighted previously, the teams should discuss their respective input into each patient at the start of the list to ensure that the plans are compatible.

This dialogue should continue throughout the case—if difficulties occur in the anaesthetic, the surgeons should be made aware promptly. For example, unexpected hypotension and tachycardia may herald covert blood loss that the surgeons can investigate further.

The theatre environment can make a big difference to the ease of communication between teams, so music should not be so loud as to impair discussion, and, if critical events occur, it should switched off entirely. Similarly, although a screen between the head of the patient and the surgical field is often desirable, it should not be placed such that the anaesthetist cannot talk to the surgeons or view the operating site.

3.5.4 **Handover to recovery**

The handover to recovery is an important step in the patient's theatre journey. The patient should not be taken to recovery until they are maintaining their own airway (or have a patent LMA *in situ*), have good spontaneous respiratory effort, and are cardiovascularly stable, and there is a plan in place for post-operative management.

Many different models for handover exist, but at a minimum should include: name and age of patient, their relevant past medical history and allergies, the surgery they have undergone, the type of anaesthetic they have received (including any regional techniques performed), the analgesia and antiemesis they have already received, and plans for the management of recurring pain or nausea. Any critical events that have occurred during the time in theatre should be discussed.

The anaesthetist should conduct this handover after the patient has arrived and monitoring has been re-established.

The anaesthetist can return to theatre once the recovery staff have satisfied themselves the patient is stable, but, after the last case of the day, the anaesthetist should not leave the theatre suite until the last patient is alert and their pain is controlled.

3.6 **Self-assessment questions**

Answer either true or false for each of the following questions. The answers can be found in Appendix 2.

1. Concerning ASA grades:
   - A. An ASA 1 patient might have well-controlled asthma
   - B. If a patient had a penicillin allergy, they would be classified as ASA 2
   - C. An ASA 3 patient has a moderate systemic illness
   - D. A patient with a life-limiting illness, such as unstable angina, would be ASA 4
   - E. ASA 5 patients are at high risk of mortality

2. When conducting an airway assessment:
   - A. A Mallampati II view implies that the uvula and tonsils are partially visible and the hard and soft palates can both be seen easily
   - B. A patient with Mallampati score of IV would be suitable for an RSI
   - C. Thyromental distance is measured with the patient relaxed and the head in a neutral position
   - D. Edentulous patients have airways that are potentially difficult to manage
   - E. The presence of a beard predicts difficult intubation

3. A 32-year-old woman presents for elective hysteroscopy. She has previously undergone uneventful general anaesthesia for elective procedures. She has no

previous medical history and is allergic to penicillin. Which of the following investigations would be appropriate in this patient?

A. ECG
B. Biochemistry
C. Full blood count
D. Coagulation
E. Chest X-ray

4. **Assuming the airway assessment was reassuring, which techniques for managing her airway would be appropriate?**

A. Routine induction with propofol, followed by insertion of an LMA
B. Routine induction with propofol, followed by insertion of a tracheal tube
C. Inhalational induction with sevoflurane, followed by insertion of a tracheal tube
D. RSI with sodium thiopental, followed by insertion of a tracheal tube
E. Routine induction with propofol, followed by maintenance by face mask

5. **Which of the following maintenance techniques would be appropriate for this patient?**

A. Oxygen, air, and sevoflurane
B. Oxygen, nitrous oxide, and isoflurane
C. Oxygen, air, and desflurane
D. Oxygen, air, and propofol TIVA
E. Air and sevoflurane

6. **Which of the following would feature in the post-operative analgesic plan for this patient?**

A. Paracetamol 1 g qds
B. IV morphine PCA
C. Codeine phosphate 30 mg qds
D. Ibuprofen 400 mg qds
E. IM morphine 10 mg hourly

7. **A 64-year-old patient presents with small bowel obstruction secondary to adhesions and needs an emergency laparotomy. He has previously undergone uneventful general anaesthesia for elective procedures. He has a background of hypertension treated with atenolol and is otherwise well. He has no allergies. Which of the following investigations would be appropriate in this patient?**

A. ECG
B. Biochemistry
C. Full blood count

D. Coagulation
E. Chest X-ray

8. **Assuming the airway assessment was reassuring, which induction technique would be appropriate for this patient?**

    A. Routine induction with propofol, followed by insertion of an LMA
    B. Routine induction with propofol, followed by insertion of a tracheal tube
    C. Inhalational induction with sevoflurane, followed by insertion of a tracheal tube
    D. RSI with sodium thiopental, followed by insertion of a tracheal tube
    E. Routine induction with propofol, followed by maintenance by face mask

9. **Which of the following maintenance techniques would be appropriate for this patient?**

    A. Oxygen, air, and sevoflurane
    B. Oxygen, nitrous oxide, and isoflurane
    C. Oxygen, air, and desflurane
    D. Oxygen, air, and propofol TIVA
    E. Air and sevoflurane

10. **Which of the following would feature in the post-operative analgesic plan for this patient?**

    A. Paracetamol 1 g qds
    B. IV morphine PCA
    C. Codeine phosphate 30 mg qds
    D. Ibuprofen 400 mg qds
    E. IM morphine 10 mg hourly

Chapter 4

Routine induction of general anaesthesia

4.1 Introduction

In an average year, an anaesthetist will give several hundreds of anaesthetics. Most are routine, but not all critical events can be predicted, and, before every case, the anaesthetist must carefully plan and prepare for the unexpected.

4.2 Routine induction of general anaesthesia

Routine induction of anaesthesia describes non-'rapid sequence' techniques. It usually refers to induction in fasted patients. Most commonly, propofol is the induction agent of choice, although other agents, including sevoflurane, are an option under certain circumstances.

4.2.1 Preparing the anaesthetic room

Before the patient arrives, the anaesthetic machine should be checked, according to AAGBI guidelines (see Section 1.5), and the location of emergency and resuscitation equipment should be confirmed. The team should be briefed with regard to the anaesthetic plan (see Section 3.5).

Draw up the necessary drugs and any emergency drugs that you may require. Most routine anaesthetics will use a combination of an induction agent, a short-acting opioid, an antiemetic, and a muscle relaxant if appropriate. Suxamethonium, atropine, ephedrine, and metaraminol will often be drawn up and the syringes capped for use, if needed.

A typical drug tray for an ASA 1 or 2 patient undergoing intermediate surgery with a tracheal tube might include:

- 20 mL propofol 1% (200 mg)
- 2 mL fentanyl 50 micrograms/mL (100 micrograms)
- 5 mL atracurium 10 mg/mL (50 mg)
- 2 mL dexamethasone 4 mg/mL (8 mg)
- Antibiotics, as indicated by local protocol.

And placed to one side:

- 10 mL ephedrine 3 mg/mL (30 mg)
- 20 mL metaraminol 0.5 mg/mL (10 mg)

- 2 mL suxamethonium 50 mg/mL (100 mg)*
- 2 mL atropine 300 micrograms/mL (600 micrograms).

* Kept in the refrigerator.

4.2.2 **Preparing the patient**

When the patient arrives, the WHO sign-in checks must be completed (see Section 3.5.1). Next, establish monitoring (ECG, NIBP, and oxygen saturations), and gain IV access. Ensure the patient is properly positioned for airway maintenance and that the trolley is at an appropriate height.

Consider any alternative steps that might be required in the event of airway difficulties.

4.2.3 **Induction**

Preoxygenate the patient using high-flow oxygen from the anaesthetic circuit, and, when ready, administer the induction agent (e.g. 2 mg/kg propofol). It is often desirable to use a 'coinduction agent'. This is usually either a rapidly acting opioid or a benzodiazepine. Typically, this results in a smoother induction and a reduction in the sympathetic response observed during airway manipulation. If a coinduction agent is used, it should be given time to reach clinical effect before the induction agent is given (usually several minutes).

Once the patient is asleep, check that mask ventilation is possible. If so, introduce the maintenance agent (e.g. isoflurane). If an LMA is required, it can be inserted now. If a tracheal tube is planned, give the muscle relaxant at this point (e.g. atracurium 0.5 mg/kg), and wait the required time for it to reach its effect. Perform direct laryngoscopy, and insert the tube.

Once the airway is placed, perform a series of manual breaths to check it is correctly sited, and commence mechanical ventilation if a muscle relaxant has been used.

Keep the patient breathing 100% oxygen until transferred into theatre.

4.2.4 **Transfer to theatre**

Disconnect the monitoring equipment first, leaving the breathing circuit the last thing to be detached. Move the patient promptly to theatre, and first reconnect the breathing circuit, ensuring that oxygen is flowing and the vaporizer has been turned on. If connecting to an anaesthetic machine with a circle breathing system, initial settings of 4 L/min oxygen would be appropriate. The volatile of choice should be started, but care should be taken not to start at too high a level, particularly since both isoflurane and desflurane are irritant to the respiratory tract in light planes of anaesthesia. Suitable vaporizer settings for isoflurane might be 2% or for sevoflurane around 4% (sevoflurane is half as potent as isoflurane, and therefore twice the concentration is required).

Perform one or two manual breaths to ensure the circuit is patent and there are no leaks. Confirm ventilation by checking chest movement and capnography. Turn on the mechanical ventilator, if required, ensuring that an appropriate tidal volume is being delivered and that airway pressures are acceptable.

Monitoring should be reconnected as soon as possible, beginning with the saturation probe. If the patient will be transferred from the trolley to the operating table promptly it is acceptable to transfer before full monitoring has been established, although oxygen saturations should be measured.

With monitoring connected, ensure that NIBPs are being measured automatically and at suitable intervals. At this stage, the F_iO_2 can be reduced by introducing the second gas (air or nitrous oxide). Appropriate flow rates might be 2 L/min oxygen, 2 L/min air.

At this stage, the WHO time out can be conducted.

As it takes time for agent levels to build up in the circle, the total flow rate should continue at 4 L/min until 1 MAC end-tidal agent has been achieved, and then total flows can be gradually reduced to around 1 L. As total flow rate is reduced, the vaporizer setting will need to be increased, so the end-tidal agent concentration must be observed carefully and controls adjusted to ensure that 1 MAC is maintained.

The surgeon must check that the anaesthetist is happy before commencing the operation. It is sensible to perform a final check of the following settings before agreeing:

- Check flowmeter, SpO_2, and F_iO_2 values
- Check ventilation (tidal volume, frequency, and airway pressures) and E_tCO_2 values
- Check vaporizer setting and end-tidal agent concentration
- Check heart rate and blood pressure.

Provided these checks are satisfactory, surgery can begin.

4.3 Self-assessment questions

Answer either true or false for each of the following questions. The answers can be found in Appendix 2.

1. A 70 kg 76-year-old female presents for an elective laparoscopic cholecystectomy. She is fit and well, is a non-smoker, and has no allergies. She is appropriately fasted. It has been decided the patient should be intubated for the procedure, and her airway assessment is reassuring. Which of the following drugs are likely to be required at induction?

A. Propofol, at a dose of around 140 mg
B. Propofol, at a dose of around 200 mg
C. Sodium thiopental, at a dose of around 375 mg
D. Suxamethonium, at a dose of 100 mg
E. Glycopyrrolate, at a dose of 200 mg

2. Which of the following details are confirmed at the WHO sign-in check?

A. The patient's fasting state
B. The operation site
C. The patient's state of dentition
D. The patient's allergy status
E. The signature on the consent form

3. **The patient has no past history of PONV. Which of the following statements are true?**

   A. No antiemesis required for this case
   B. A single dose of dexamethasone should be given prior to induction
   C. A single dose of dexamethasone should be given after induction
   D. She is at very high risk of post-operative nausea, so a TIVA technique should be used
   E. Ondansetron would be suitable for post-operative use

4. **If a coinduction agent, such as 100 micrograms fentanyl or 2 mg midazolam, is desired, when is the most appropriate time to give it to this patient?**

   A. As soon as the patient arrives in the anaesthetic room to reduce anxiety
   B. As soon as the cannula has been put in, but before the monitoring has been established
   C. As soon as monitoring has been established
   D. Immediately before the induction agent is administered
   E. Immediately after the induction agent is administered

5. **Which of the following monitoring should be applied before starting the anaesthetic?**

   A. NIBP
   B. ECG
   C. Pulse oximetry
   D. Peripheral nerve stimulator
   E. Temperature

6. **Which of the following muscle relaxants and doses would be appropriate for this patient?**

   A. 50 mg atracurium
   B. 100 mg rocuronium
   C. 7 mg vecuronium
   D. 100 mg suxamethonium
   E. 40 mg rocuronium

7. **Which of the following can be used to check the tracheal tube position?**

   A. Capnography waveform
   B. Auscultation in the mid-clavicular line
   C. Auscultation in the mid-axillary line
   D. Auscultation over the stomach
   E. Misting of the tracheal tube

8. **The patient's blood pressure drops from 160/95 to 90/50 after induction and intubation. Her heart rate is 70. Which of the following statements are true?**

   A. No treatment is required at this stage. The blood pressure should be rechecked in 5 min
   B. Treatment is required. Ephedrine 6 mg would be appropriate
   C. Treatment is required. A fluid challenge with Hartmann's solution would be appropriate
   D. Treatment is required. Metaraminol 6 mg would be appropriate
   E. Treatment is required. Glycopyrrolate 200 mg would be appropriate

9. **The patient is transferred to theatre and connected to the circle system on the anaesthetic machine. What would be appropriate initial settings for the anaesthetic machine?**

   A. FGFs of 400 mL/min oxygen and 400 mL/min nitrous oxide
   B. FGFs of 2 L/min oxygen and 2 L/min air
   C. Switch the ventilator on, with a tidal volume of around 600 mL
   D. Switch on the isoflurane at 4%
   E. Switch on the sevoflurane at 4%

10. **An unexpected airway problem develops at the end of the case. Where would you be most likely to find suxamethonium quickly?**

   A. In the controlled drug cupboard
   B. In the general drug cupboard
   C. On the emergency trolley with the defibrillator
   D. In the refrigerator in an ampoule
   E. In the refrigerator already drawn up

Chapter 5

The rapid sequence induction

5.1 Introduction

The RSI is necessary for patients at risk of aspiration at induction. The risks of airway difficulties are higher than with a routine induction, and the anaesthetist must be well prepared to manage these.

5.2 The rapid sequence induction

RSI of anaesthesia describes the technique used to induce anaesthesia, muscle relaxation, and securing of the airway in the shortest possible time. A choice of either propofol or thiopental is appropriate.

It is generally performed in the non-fasted patient in whom there is a risk of aspiration, as airway reflexes are abolished by the anaesthetic. It aims to take the awake patient, who is protecting their own airway, and render them unconscious with a secured (intubated) airway in the shortest duration, thus minimizing the time interval in which aspiration may occur. It is also designed to allow the patient to wake quickly in the event of an unexpectedly difficult intubation.

5.2.1 Preparing the anaesthetic room

Before the patient arrives, the anaesthetic machine should be checked according to AAGBI guidelines (see Section 1.5), and the location of emergency and resuscitation equipment should be confirmed. The team should be briefed with regard to the anaesthetic plan (see Section 3.5).

Draw up the necessary drugs and any emergency drugs that you may require. Most RSI anaesthetics will use only an induction agent and a fast acting muscle relaxant (eg suxamethonium). Other drugs, such as fentanyl, may be needed, but should not be given until the airway has been secured. Emergency drugs such as atropine, ephedrine, and metaraminol would be drawn up and the syringes capped for use later, if needed.

A typical drug tray for an ASA 1 or 2 patient undergoing intermediate surgery might include:

- 20 mL propofol 1% (200 mg) **or** 20 mL thiopental 25 mg/mL (500 mg)
- 2 mL suxamethonium 50 mg/mL (100 mg).

And placed to one side:

- 2 mL fentanyl 50 micrograms/mL (100 micrograms)
- 5 mL atracurium 10 mg/mL (50 mg)
- 2 mL dexamethasone 4 mg/mL (8 mg)
- Antibiotics, as indicated by local protocol
- 10 mL ephedrine 3 mg/mL (30 mg)
- 20 mL metaraminol 0.5 mg/mL (10 mg)
- 2 mL suxamethonium 50 mg/mL (100 mg)*
- 2 mL atropine 300 micrograms/mL (600 micrograms).

* Kept in the refrigerator; separate from the planned induction dose.

Keeping the induction drugs separate from the other 'routine' agents during the RSI can help to minimize the risk of accidentally giving the wrong drug at a crucial moment.

5.2.2 **Preparing the patient**

When the patient arrives, the WHO Sign In checks must be completed (see Section 3.5.1). Next, establish monitoring (ECG, NIBP, and oxygen saturations), and gain IV access. Ensure the patient is properly positioned for airway maintenance and that the trolley is at an appropriate height.

Consider what alternative steps will be required in the event of airway difficulties; this is even more crucial during an RSI.

Ensure that the trolley can be placed in a head-down position, if required. Turn on the anaesthetic machine's suction device, and place the Yankauer sucker under the patient's pillow so that it can easily be reached.

5.2.3 **Induction**

Preoxygenate the patient using high-flow oxygen from the anaesthetic circuit for a full 3 min.

When ready, confirm that the assistant is ready and happy to administer cricoid pressure, then administer the induction agent (e.g. 2 mg/kg propofol or 3–7 mg/kg thiopental; see Table 5.1) and the muscle relaxant (suxamethonium 1.5 mg/kg) together. Suxamethonium crystallizes when added directly to thiopental, so the drugs should be given into a running drip, although it will be necessary to occlude it briefly when the drugs are actually given to ensure the drugs do not track up the giving set towards the fluid bag.

Coinduction agents are usually not appropriate during an RSI, so, except under unusual circumstances, fentanyl or midazolam should not be given prior to induction. They may be given once the airway is secured. This ensures that the patient can be woken rapidly in the event of airway difficulties.

Once the patient is asleep, do not perform mask ventilation. This increases the risk of gastric inflation and regurgitation. After the suxamethonium has taken effect (30–45 s or after fasciculations have subsided), perform direct laryngoscopy and insert the tube.

Once the airway is placed, perform a series of manual breaths to confirm correct placement, checking the capnograph and chest movement, then commence mechanical ventilation. Turn on the vaporizer (e.g. isoflurane at 1–2%).

Keep the patient breathing 100% oxygen until transferred into theatre.

Table 5.1 Comparison of propofol and sodium thiopental	
Propofol	Thiopental
Dose: 2 mg/kg	Dose: 3–7 mg/kg
Onset time: 45 s	Onset time: 30 s
Duration of action: 5–10 min	Duration of action: 5–10 min
Propofol is commonly used for RSI, as it is a drug with which all anaesthetists are highly familiar. It has a slower onset time than thiopental, but possibly a slightly shorter duration of action. The dose–response to propofol may be slightly less predictable than thiopental.	Thiopental is classically the 'agent of choice' for RSI, but its use is becoming less common. It may be more predictable than propofol and has a faster onset time, although longer duration of action. It has fewer cardiovascular effects than equivalent doses of propofol. Thiopental is contraindicated in patients with porphyria and can cause significant tissue damage if it extravasates or is injected intra-arterially.

5.2.4 **Transfer to theatre**

Disconnect monitoring equipment first, leaving the breathing circuit the last thing to be detached. Move the patient promptly into theatre, and first reconnect the breathing circuit, ensuring that oxygen is flowing and the vaporizer has been turned on. If connecting to an anaesthetic machine with a circle breathing system, initial settings of 4 L/min oxygen and 2% isoflurane would be an appropriate start.

Perform one or two manual breaths to ensure the circuit is patent and there are no leaks. Confirm ventilation by checking chest movement and capnography. Turn on the mechanical ventilator, if required, ensuring that an appropriate tidal volume is being delivered and that airway pressures are acceptable.

Monitoring should be reconnected as soon as possible, beginning with the saturation probe. If the patient will be transferred from the trolley to the operating table promptly, it is acceptable to transfer before full monitoring has been established, although oxygen saturations should be measured.

With monitoring connected, ensure that NIBPs are being measured automatically and at suitable intervals. At this stage, the F_iO_2 can be reduced by introducing the second gas (air or nitrous oxide). Appropriate settings might be 2 L/min oxygen, 2 L/min air, and 2% isoflurane.

At this stage, the WHO time out can be conducted.

As it takes time for agent levels to build up in the circle, the total flow rate should continue at 4 L/min until 1 MAC end-tidal agent has been achieved, and then total flows can be gradually reduced to around 1 L. As total flow rate is reduced, the vaporizer setting will need to be increased, so the end-tidal agent concentration must be observed carefully and controls adjusted to ensure that 1 MAC is maintained.

The duration of suxamethonium is typically 5–10 min, so a long-acting muscle relaxant (e.g. atracurium) is often required. The long-acting relaxant should not be given until the suxamethonium has worn off. This can be checked with a nerve stimulator or by waiting until the patient shows signs of recovery from neuromuscular blockade such as starting to make their own respiratory effort.

The surgeon must check that the anaesthetist is happy before commencing the operation. It is sensible to perform a final check of the following settings before agreeing:

- Check flowmeter, SpO_2, and F_iO_2 values
- Check ventilation (tidal volume, frequency, and airway pressures) and E_tCO_2 values
- Check vaporizer setting and end-tidal agent concentration
- Check heart rate and blood pressure.

Provided these checks are satisfactory, surgery can begin.

5.3 Self-assessment questions

Answer either true or false for each of the following questions. The answers can be found in Appendix 2.

1. An 85 kg 32-year-old male presents for a laparoscopic appendectomy. He has well-controlled asthma but tolerates NSAIDs. He is a non-smoker and has no allergies. He last ate 6 h ago. It has been decided the patient should have an RSI. The airway assessment is reassuring. What drugs will be most appropriate for induction?

   A. 450 mg sodium thiopental
   B. 100 mg rocuronium
   C. 100 micrograms fentanyl
   D. 50 mg atracurium
   E. 125 mg suxamethonium

2. Which of the following preparations are required for a patient requiring an RSI?

   A. Position the airway in the 'sniffing the morning air' position
   B. Ask a third member of staff to be in the anaesthetic room with you
   C. Place a nasogastric (NG) tube to aspirate gastric contents
   D. Locate the cricoid cartilage
   E. Flush the IV cannula before beginning

3. What is the most appropriate sequence of actions when performing an RSI?

   A. Position patient; activate suction; preoxygenate for 3 min; give induction agent, then muscle relaxant; intubate
   B. Position patient; preoxygenate for 3 min; give induction agent; activate suction; give muscle relaxant; intubate
   C. Position patient; activate suction; preoxygenate for 3 min; give induction agent; face mask-ventilate; give muscle relaxant; intubate
   D. Preoxygenate for 3 min; position patient; activate suction; give induction agent, then muscle relaxant; intubate
   E. Preoxygenate for 3 min; activate suction; give induction agent, then muscle relaxant; position patient; intubate

4. Which of the following are potential risks when using suxamethonium?
   A. Hyperkalaemia
   B. Bradycardia
   C. Raised ICP
   D. MH
   E. Anaphylaxis

5. Which of the following are true about cricoid pressure?
   A. Application of force on the cricoid occludes the oesophagus
   B. The technique is also called the Sellick manoeuvre
   C. It can only be released when instructed by the anaesthetist
   D. It protects the airway against soiling if the patient vomits
   E. It cannot be released, even if the laryngoscopy view is poor

6. Thiopental is presented as a powder containing 500 mg. It is usually mixed up to give a 20 mL solution. Which of the following statements are true?
   A. Mixing 500 mg into 20 mL yields a 25% solution
   B. A 55 kg patient would require a dose of around 275 mg
   C. 11 mL of thiopental would be required to give a dose of 275 mg
   D. Thiopental is incompatible with suxamethonium
   E. Thiopental is titrated to effect during RSI

7. Assuming an otherwise fit patient, when is the most appropriate time to give a coinduction agent, such as 100 micrograms fentanyl or 2 mg midazolam, during RSI?
   A. As soon as the patient arrives in the anaesthetic room, to reduce anxiety
   B. Prior to starting preoxygenation
   C. Immediately before the induction agent is administered
   D. Immediately after the induction agent is administered
   E. It is not appropriate to give a coinduction agent

8. When would it be appropriate to give a long-acting muscle relaxant (such as atracurium) after an RSI?
   A. Immediately following the suxamethonium
   B. As soon as the tracheal tube is secured
   C. On transfer to theatre
   D. On noticing irregularity on the capnograph trace
   E. After checking with a peripheral nerve stimulator

9. What would be an appropriate choice of maintenance technique after an RSI?

A. Propofol
B. Thiopental
C. Sevoflurane
D. Isoflurane
E. Desflurane

10. The 85 kg patient is transferred to theatre and connected to the circle system on the anaesthetic machine. What would be appropriate initial settings?

A. FGFs of 2 L/min oxygen and 2 L/min air
B. Switch the ventilator on, with a tidal volume of around 575 mL
C. Set the ventilator at a respiratory rate of 12
D. Switch on desflurane at 12%
E. Switch on isoflurane at 2%

Chapter 6

Central neuraxial blockade

6.1 Introduction

Central neuraxial blocks, such as spinal or epidural anaesthesia, are useful and commonly practised techniques with which the junior anaesthetist will become familiar in their early training.

6.2 Central neuraxial blockade

Central neuraxial blockade is a term that describes spinal and epidural anaesthesia. Both techniques can produce dense regional blocks of the trunk and lower limbs, making them suitable for anaesthesia in a wide range of orthopaedic, urological, and obstetric procedures. Drug doses, onset, duration, and pattern of block differ, depending upon which technique is used.

In addition to their role as anaesthetic techniques in their own right, central neuraxial blocks can provide excellent analgesia post-operatively and reduce or abolish the stress response associated with surgery.

Functioning central blocks provide excellent pain relief and respiratory function post-operatively. The improvement in respiratory mechanics, afforded by better pain relief and the avoidance of sedative drugs like propofol or opioids, particularly benefits patients with severe respiratory comorbidities. There is, however, no clear mortality benefit to undergoing surgery using a neuraxial technique in the general surgical population.

Central neuraxial techniques are very commonly used to provide anaesthesia for women undergoing surgical procedures in labour, typically Caesarean section, manual removal of placenta, or for forceps deliveries. General anaesthesia in late pregnancy requires a rapid sequence induction (see Section 5.2), as pregnancy confers a significant risk of aspiration, but the incidence of difficult (and failed) intubation (see Section 7.2) is much higher in the obstetric population. Wherever possible, avoidance of general anaesthesia in late pregnancy is highly desirable.

These techniques cannot be performed in patients with a risk of bleeding or those with sepsis in whom a bacteraemia may result in a spinal or epidural abscess.

6.2.1 Anatomy of the spinal cord

In adults, the spinal cord begins at the foramen magnum and terminates at the L1–L2 vertebrae. The spinal cord is covered by the meninges, which continue below the spinal cord to terminate in the conus in the sacrum. Between L1–L2 and the conus, the meninges contain CSF and spinal nerves.

The epidural space is a potential space that lies between the outer surface of the meninges and the vertebral bodies anteriorly and the laminae posteriorly. The epidural space contains epidural fat, epidural veins, and nerve roots as they leave the meninges to exit the vertebral column.

6.2.2 **Spinal anaesthesia**

Spinal techniques are usually performed to provide surgical anaesthesia for short- or medium-duration operations on the lower body. They are occasionally combined with general anaesthesia.

Spinal anaesthetics are usually placed by performing an injection at the level of L3–4 or L4–5. Above these levels, there is a risk of trauma to the spinal cord, whereas, below these levels lie the fused vertebrae of the sacrum. A 'spinal' can be placed in either a sitting or lateral position, with the patient curled forward. This is a sterile technique; the anaesthetist must be scrubbed and gowned.

Spinal needles, such as the Whitacre needle (see Fig 6.1), are designed with 'atraumatic' pencil-point tips. These part the fibres of dural membrane, rather than cut them. This reduces the risk of a persisting hole in the dura through which CSF could leak, causing a post-dural puncture headache (PDPH). They are usually small needles of 25–27G.

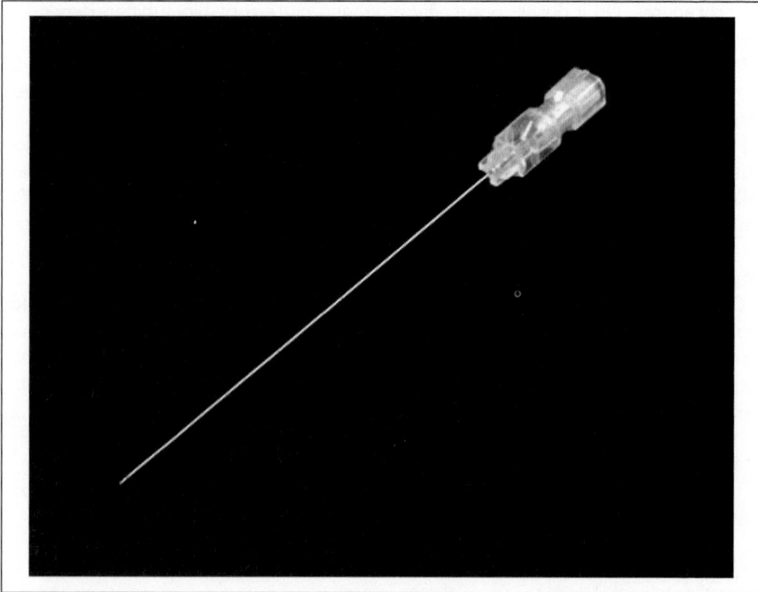

Fig 6.1 A Whitacre needle used for spinal anaesthesia. The needle is narrow (25G) and has a pencil-point tip designed to minimize the risk of PDPH. A stylet occupies the centre of the needle during insertion to minimize the transfer of tissue into the spine and must be removed prior to injection.

Typically, 'heavy' solutions of LA are used (see Section 2.8.2). These are mixtures of an LA, usually bupivacaine 0.5% and 8% glucose. Heavy solutions are hyperbaric compared to CSF, meaning they sink under gravity. Positioning of the patient head up or head down can therefore be used to control the speed and height of the block as it develops. Lipid-soluble opioids, like fentanyl (see Section 2.6.3.2) or diamorphine, may be added to the LA to improve the quality of block.

Spinal anaesthesia takes 10–15 min to develop. Although variable and dependent on the drugs and doses used, surgical anaesthesia typically lasts for around 90 min. It takes several hours for the motor and sensory block to completely subside.

A spinal anaesthetic provides complete sensory loss below a certain spinal level. The patient should lose light and deep touch, pain, temperature, and proprioception, as well as experience profound motor block. 'Block height' refers to the dermatome representing the maximum extent of the block. Block height is usually measured using either ice or ethyl-chloride spray (which feels ice-cold to touch).

Landmarks for assessing block height can be seen in Fig 6.2. The block needs to be high enough to affect all nerves supplying the surgical site. A Caesarian section requires an incision in the lower abdomen below the umbilicus; however, a block that only reached the level of the umbilicus would be inadequate, and the patient would feel pain. This is because the nerves that innervate the uterus arise from T10, while the peritoneum is innervated from as high as T4. Loss of light touch and temperature sensation to around T4 is required for Caesarean section, although much lower blocks are required for most orthopaedic or urological procedures.

6.2.3 **Epidural anaesthesia and analgesia**

From a practical perspective, there is no difference between epidural analgesia and anaesthesia; the same equipment is used to place the same catheter in the same place. The techniques differ in the drugs used and the effect sought.

Epidural anaesthesia describes using high concentration and volume of LAs to provide a sufficiently dense block to permit surgery. Epidural analgesia uses lower-strength solutions, resulting in less sensory or motor disturbance, to provide pain relief during labour or following an operation. Opioids may be added to the LA component to improve block quality.

Unlike spinals, which block all segments below a certain level, epidurals provide segmental blocks that cover only certain dermatomes. This means epidural blocks have both a maximum and minimum extent. For optimal function, an epidural should be sited at a level that corresponds to the centre of the area that should be blocked; for major (general surgical) abdominal operations, an epidural might be placed at T10 level, corresponding with innervation to the umbilicus at the centre of a laparotomy incision. Given that the spinal cord is present at this level, there is a risk of trauma, so the junior anaesthetist would not be expected to perform this technique unsupervised.

In obstetric practice, epidurals are sited at the L3–4 or L4–5 level in a position comparable to 'spinals'; this provides an optimum balance between safety, ease of insertion, and effect.

An epidural is sited using a 16G or 18G Tuohy needle (see Fig 6.3). This is a specially designed blunt needle, shaped like a spoon, with centimetre markings that help the anaesthetist to calculate the depth of the epidural space. The epidural space is located using a 'loss-of-resistance' technique whereby a saline-filled syringe is attached to the Tuohy needle and pressure applied to the plunger. While the needle tip is in tissue, this pressure

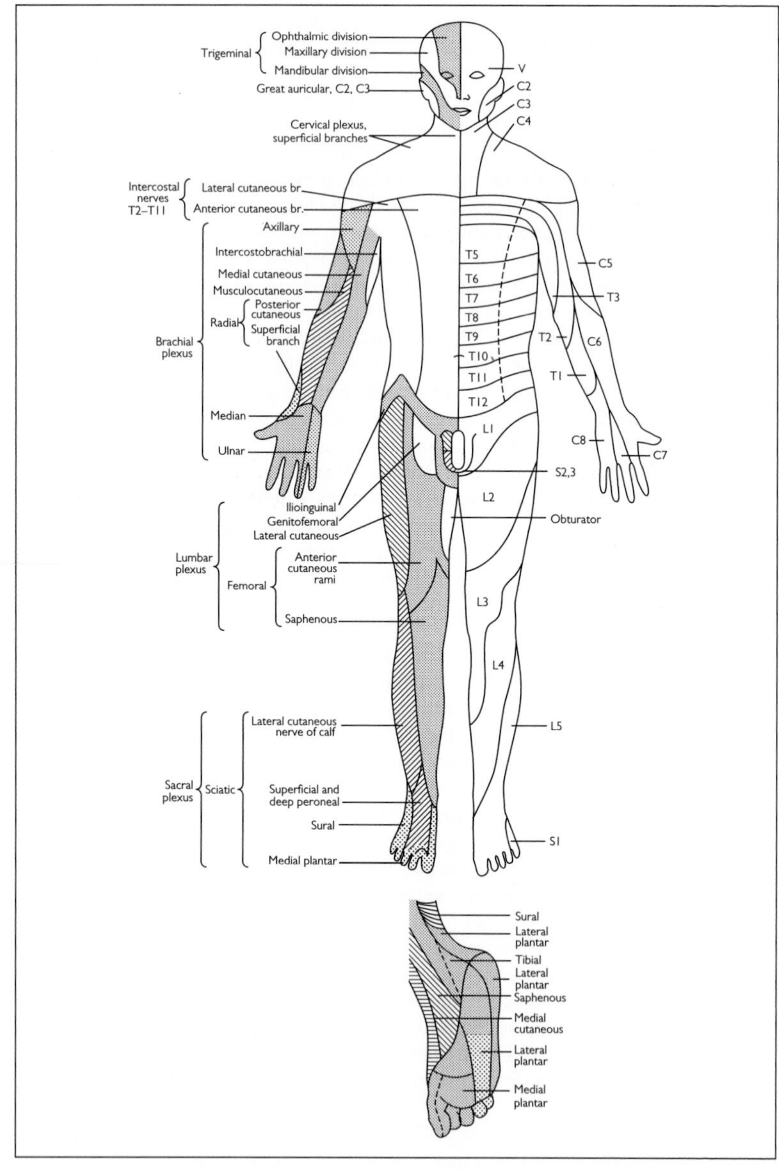

Fig 6.2 An illustrated diagram showing the landmarks that can be used to assess block height during spinal or epidural anaesthesia. Typically, a block should be at T4–5 for Caesarean section (around the level of the nipples).

Reproduced from Allman and Wilson, Oxford Handbook of Anaesthesia 3rd edition, 2011, page 1188 with permission from Oxford University Press.

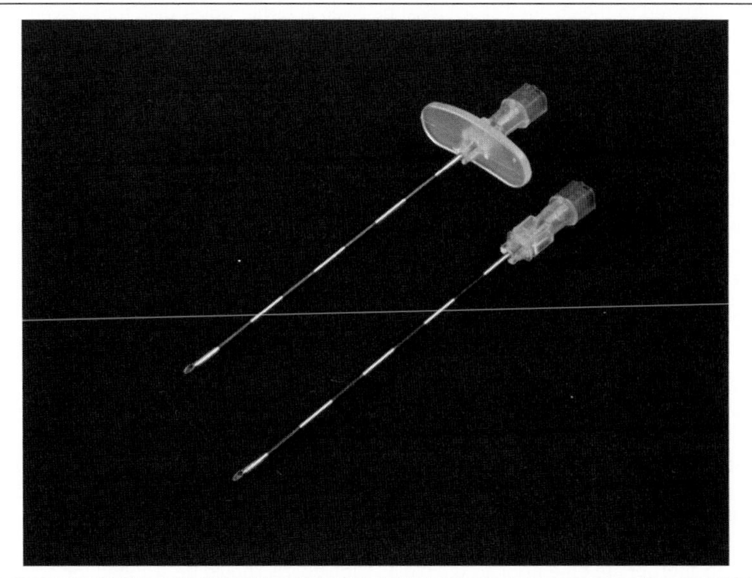

Fig 6.3 The Tuohy needle is used for insertion of epidurals. The stripes along the barrel of the needle denote centimetres from the tip of the needle and are used to help judge the depth of the epidural space from the skin. A stylet must be removed from the needle before the epidural catheter can be inserted.
Reproduced with kind permission of Becton, Dickinson and Company.

is transmitted to the needle, causing it to advance. When the tip enters the epidural space, the resistance is lost, and, instead of the pressure advancing the syringe further, the saline is simply evacuated, ensuring the needle should advance no further. So long as there is no pressure applied directly to the needle, this minimizes the risk of the needle advancing too far and inadvertently puncturing the dura. An accidental dural puncture with a large-bore Tuohy needle is called a dural tap and is a major risk factor for PDPH.

Once the epidural space is located by the loss of resistance, the anaesthetist should note the depth at which it was found, using the centimetre markings on the needle. The syringe is removed and the catheter, which must be flushed with saline prior to use, is threaded through the centre of the Tuohy needle. The needle is then carefully removed, leaving the catheter in place. The catheter also has centimetre markings on it, and its position can be adjusted to ensure that only 3–5 cm length is left inside the epidural space.

A dressing is applied to secure the catheter in position. Before use, the epidural must be aspirated to ensure neither CSF (indicating a dural tap) nor blood (indicating an intravascular placement) is present. A test-dose of LA can then be administered.

Negative aspiration does not fully exclude a dural tap, so the first dose given should not exceed a standard spinal dose of LA. If, after 5–10 min, the patient experiences no sensory or motor change, then a full epidural dose can be administered. Drugs administered to the epidural space must be given at higher doses than those given spinally and take longer to work. A typical spinal for Caesarean section might require 2.5 mL of 0.5% heavy bupivacaine, whereas 20 mL of 0.5% bupivacaine might be required to produce an equivalent block using an epidural. Epidural anaesthesia can take up to 30 min to develop.

After insertion, an epidural can remain *in situ* for up to 3–4 days, during which it may be connected to an infusion device to deliver continuous analgesia. This is usually patient-controlled epidural analgesia (PCEA) that combines continuous infusion with patient-triggered boluses. If a patient is receiving fentanyl or diamorphine through an epidural, they should not simultaneously receive strong opioids by another route, as there is risk of respiratory depression.

6.2.4 **Anticoagulation and neuraxial blockade**

Although it is generally considered safe to perform a spinal or epidural in patients receiving low-dose aspirin treatment (75 mg once daily), these techniques are absolutely contraindicated in patients with a coagulopathy or thrombocytopenia. Absolute limits vary from unit to unit, but generally the junior anaesthetist should not perform a spinal or epidural in a patient with a platelet count <100 or an international normalized ratio (INR) >1.2. If there is any doubt, consult with a senior colleague before proceeding.

In patients receiving antiplatelet or anticoagulant therapy, drugs must be stopped for an appropriate time prior to the block. Clopidogrel should be stopped for at least 7 days beforehand. Prophylactic LMWHs should not have been administered in the last 12 h (24 h for treatment dose), and patients receiving warfarin should not undergo a neuraxial blockade until the INR has normalized.

Consideration must be taken as to timing the removal of an epidural catheter with regard to anticoagulant doses; it is recommended that the catheter is not removed until 12 h after a prophylactic LMWH dose, and any subsequent dose should not be given within 4 h of catheter removal. It is safe to give prophylaxis doses of LMWH while the epidural is *in situ*.

6.2.5 **Complications of neuraxial blockade**

Serious adverse effects from neuraxial blockade are rare, but there are common side effects for which the anaesthetist must be prepared.

6.2.5.1 *Neurological effects*

- Both spinal and epidural anaesthesia produce motor block, alongside the sensory block. Although nearly complete with spinal blocks, the degree to which motor function is affected by epidural blocks is largely a function of the concentration of LA used; with high-dose 0.5% bupivacaine (e.g. for a Caesarean section), the motor block may be very similar to a spinal; however, with lower-strength mixtures, e.g. 0.1% bupivacaine used for PCEA, the patient might be expected to mobilize almost normally
- An excessively high block from an epidural may reach C1, with widespread motor and autonomic effects; however, as the epidural space terminates at the skull, the LA will not reach the CNS

- Since spinal CSF spaces are continuous with intracranial CSF, it is possible for the LA dose from a spinal to reach the brain, resulting in a 'total spinal'. This causes motor and autonomic effects similar to an epidural reaching C1 but has the additional complication of intracranial LA causing disruption to cerebral function. This can manifest as confusion, agitation, convulsions, and abnormalities of conscious level
- Significant neurological damage occurs between 1:10 000 and 1:25 000 cases, depending on the patient population studied.

6.2.5.2 *Cardiovascular effects*

- Sympathetic fibres are also affected by the block, so sympathetic supply to the anaesthetized area is reduced or absent. This causes vasodilatation and venous pooling. The associated reduction in venous return, and therefore cardiac preload, can produce significant falls in blood pressure. The patient may experience sensations of nausea as blood pressure falls, and the anaesthetist should be ready to administer a suitable vasopressor. It is good practice to have a drug, such as ephedrine, drawn up and ready to administer.
- Spinal blocks develop rapidly, which can cause sudden and profound changes in blood pressure; as such, a spinal may not be appropriate in patients with significant cardiac disease and is absolutely contraindicated in fixed cardiac output states like aortic stenosis.
- If the block rises above T4, it may affect sympathetic cardio-accelerator fibres, which originate from T1 to T4. Loss of sympathetic supply to the heart results in bradycardia, and, if combined with reduced blood pressure, cardiac output may fall significantly.

6.2.5.3 *Respiratory effects*

- A high motor block will affect respiratory function, as intercostal muscles are supplied by thoracic spinal nerves. Most respiratory effort is generated by the diaphragm, innervated by nerves from C3 to C5. In healthy patients, this effect is minimally significant, although the patient may complain of subjective feelings of chest heaviness.

6.2.5.4 *Other effects*

- An opioid-containing spinal or epidural injectate can cause itching, which, in some patients, may be severe. This does not respond to antihistamines well, but naloxone may be used to treat it. This does carry the risk of reducing analgesic effectiveness.
- PDPH may result from either a spinal or an epidural that has caused an inadvertent dural puncture. The risk of dural puncture is associated with the size of the needle and the design of the tip; smaller needles with pencil-point tips carry lower risks than those of larger size or with cutting-type tips. Classically, dural puncture headaches are highly postural, with symptoms absent or reduced in the supine position. Treatment includes regular analgesia, avoidance of dehydration, and, in severe cases, the administration of an epidural blood-patch.

- LA toxicity (see Section 7.8) is a potential hazard of central neuraxial blockade. Most likely to occur during epidural anaesthesia where high doses of LA are required to achieve an appropriate block (e.g. Caesarean section); toxicity can also occur during spinal anaesthesia if an intravascular injection occurs. The anaesthetist must observe maximum permitted LA doses and always aspirate before injection. Protocols exist for the management of LA toxicity, and an emergency box containing lipid emulsion should be immediately available in clinical areas where high doses of LA are used.

6.2.6 **Consent for central neuraxial blockade**

Informed consent is vital to successful central neuraxial techniques. This should include a discussion of the advantages and disadvantages of the block and any procedure-specific risks.

The safest way to insert an epidural or a spinal is with the patient awake. In some rare circumstances, it can be necessary to perform such a technique on an anaesthetized patient, but this carries additional risk and is something that should only be conducted by a senior anaesthetist.

It is crucial that the awake patient is able to cooperate, as careful positioning makes siting of the block more straightforward. Before performing the technique, the patient should be told what to expect at insertion and what sensations (e.g. motor block and itch) will occur as the block develops. It should be explained that nausea may be a sign of hypotension and they should inform the anaesthetist if they start to feel nauseated.

As part of informed consent, patients should be warned of specific risks. These include:

- Motor block
- PDPH
- Temporary or permanent nerve injury
- Itch
- Shivering
- Failure of the technique
- Hypotension ± nausea.

Techniques performed around L3–4 are generally safe, but risks vary with epidurals placed at different levels.

6.3 **Self-assessment questions**

Answer either true or false for each of the following questions. The answers can be found in Appendix 2.

1. Concerning a spinal anaesthetic:

   A. The spinal cord runs from the foramen magnum to the conus in the sacrum

   B. A spinal anaesthetic can be safely performed at L3–4

   C. Heavy bupivacaine is used to control spread of the anaesthetic

D. Morphine is commonly used in spinal anaesthetics
E. Numbness should be developing by 10 min

2. **Needles for spinal anaesthesia:**

A. Are usually 18–22G
B. Quinke needles, with cutting tips, are typically used in anaesthetic practice
C. Tuohy needles can be used to puncture the dura for spinal anaesthesia
D. Spinal needles with pencil points are preferred
E. The risk of PDPH is related to the size of needle which punctures the dura

3. **Which of the following are true of spinal anaesthesia?**

A. A spinal anaesthetic produces complete sensory loss below the level of the block
B. Spinal anaesthesia disrupts autonomic innervation to the lower limbs
C. Spinal anaesthesia is the anaesthetic of choice for patients with cardiac disease
D. Spinal anaesthesia cannot be used for abdominal procedures
E. Spinal anaesthesia cannot be combined with general anaesthesia

4. **Concerning equipment needed for epidural anaesthesia:**

A. A Tuohy needle can be used to locate the epidural space
B. Epidural needles are larger than spinal needles
C. The stripes on the outside of an epidural needle are to aid identification of the equipment
D. An epidural catheter is designed to be placed just underneath the dura
E. Any syringe can be used for a loss-of-resistance technique during epidural insertion

5. **When placing an epidural:**

A. The patient should always be sitting up
B. The patient should always be awake
C. Consent is not required if the patient is in pain
D. Not more than 5 cm length of catheter should be inserted into the epidural space
E. Drug doses in an epidural are comparable with spinal anaesthesia

6. **Which of the following drugs could be administered via an epidural?**

A. Plain bupivacaine
B. Heavy bupivacaine
C. Lidocaine

D. Fentanyl
E. Diamorphine

7. **Which of the following statements about block height are true?**

A. Altered sensation to the level of the umbilicus would imply the block has reached T10
B. A block above T4 can be associated with bradycardia
C. Altered sensation at the xiphisternum suggests the block has reached T8
D. Tingling in the hands suggests that the block has reached T1
E. Sensations of chest tightness imply the block is affecting cervical nerve roots

8. **Which of the following tests would be used to check block height?**

A. Ethyl-chloride spray, to test temperature sensation
B. Ice, to test temperature sensation
C. A tuning fork, to test vibration sense
D. Cotton wool, to test light touch
E. A needle, to test pain

9. **Anticoagulation:**

A. Central neuraxial blockade cannot be performed on any patient taking aspirin therapy
B. Central neuraxial blockade cannot be performed on any patient taking clopidogrel therapy
C. DVT prophylaxis using an LMWH cannot be given to a patient with an epidural *in situ*
D. An INR should be routinely checked before inserting a labour epidural in a fit and well woman
E. An epidural catheter can be inserted into a patient 12 h after a treatment dose of dalteparin

10. **The following are recognized side effects of central neuraxial blockade:**

A. Itch
B. Nausea
C. Hypotension
D. Motor weakness
E. Headache

Chapter 7

Emergency drills

7.1 Introduction

There are a number of emergencies that can occur during anaesthesia. Some are relatively common, while some are so rare the anaesthetist may only encounter the situation once in their career. You never know if the next case will be the one to experience an emergency, and there is a need to be vigilant at all times.

7.2 Airway problems at induction

In the majority of cases, a difficult intubation can be predicted by a careful history and thorough clinical assessment prior to induction (see Section 3.2.2). Unfortunately, not all difficult intubations can be predicted, and some are therefore unanticipated. These situations are stressful, but most can be resolved by simple measures. It is important that the anaesthetist mentally prepares the 'failed intubation drill' prior to each induction so that the sequence of actions can be carried out swiftly and effectively (see Box 7.1).

7.2.1 Preventing difficult airway situations

Perhaps the most critical component of airway management is preventing unanticipated difficulty. Every patient should be carefully positioned prior to induction, with the table at an appropriate height and the head and neck placed in the 'sniffing the morning air' position, achieved by flexion of the lower cervical spine and extension of C1–C2.

All patients should be preoxygenated prior to induction. This ensures that, should difficulty occur, the maximum time is available to correct the problem. Without preoxygenation, desaturation occurs in a matter of seconds after induction, but, with proper preoxygenation, the period before desaturation can be prolonged by several minutes.

If the airway is predictably difficult, the anaesthetist must prepare. It is neither safe nor appropriate to proceed with induction and 'hope for the best'.

Box 7.1 Learning point

Remember: **failing to intubate the patient will not cause immediate harm, but failing to oxygenate them will be rapidly fatal**. If you cannot easily site the tracheal tube, focus on oxygenation by any means.

7.2.2 **Human factors and airway difficulties**

Practising and rehearsing the failed intubation drill is imperative; it ensures that all members of the anaesthetic team are unified in their approach, and can help the anaesthetic assistant to anticipate the anaesthetist's needs.

An environment that favours communication is also crucial. This means that the environment should be optimized; the room should be quiet, music should be turned off, and conversations should be kept to a minimum. There should be no disturbances to distract the team at this crucial phase.

Team dynamics also impact on communication. It is difficult to maintain situational awareness during stressful events, and members of the team should feel empowered to convey relevant information or suggestions to the anaesthetist. This might include communicating changes in oxygen saturation or the number of attempts the anaesthetist has made to intubate the patient.

One of the dangers of dealing with the difficult airway is that the focus of attention becomes completing the intubation while losing track of the situation as a whole. This is termed a fixation error (see Fig 7.1). It is imperative that the anaesthetist remembers that, in the event of airway difficulty, the priority is oxygenation by any means. Protection of the airway from aspiration and completion of the surgery are important but are secondary factors that can be addressed after oxygenation has been achieved. In most cases, especially for the less experienced anaesthetist, the safest course is to wake the patient up.

7.2.3 **Unanticipated difficult intubation during routine induction**

The guidelines published by DAS are conveniently divided into 'plans' (see Fig 7.2). These represent the sequence of actions, and their objectives, that the anaesthetist

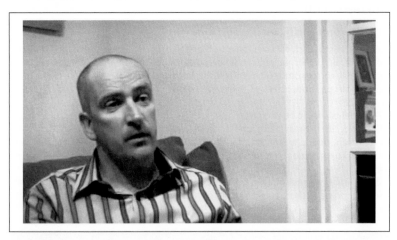

Fig 7.1 The video *Just a routine operation: human factors in patient safety* illustrates the importance of good communication and teamwork in preventing anaesthetic disasters. Elaine Bromiley died as a result of airway problems during a routine operation in March 2005. Her husband Martin Bromiley is an airline pilot with a background in human factors, and he speaks about the events that led to Elaine's death and what could be done to prevent similar deaths. A video of this is available in the video appendix.

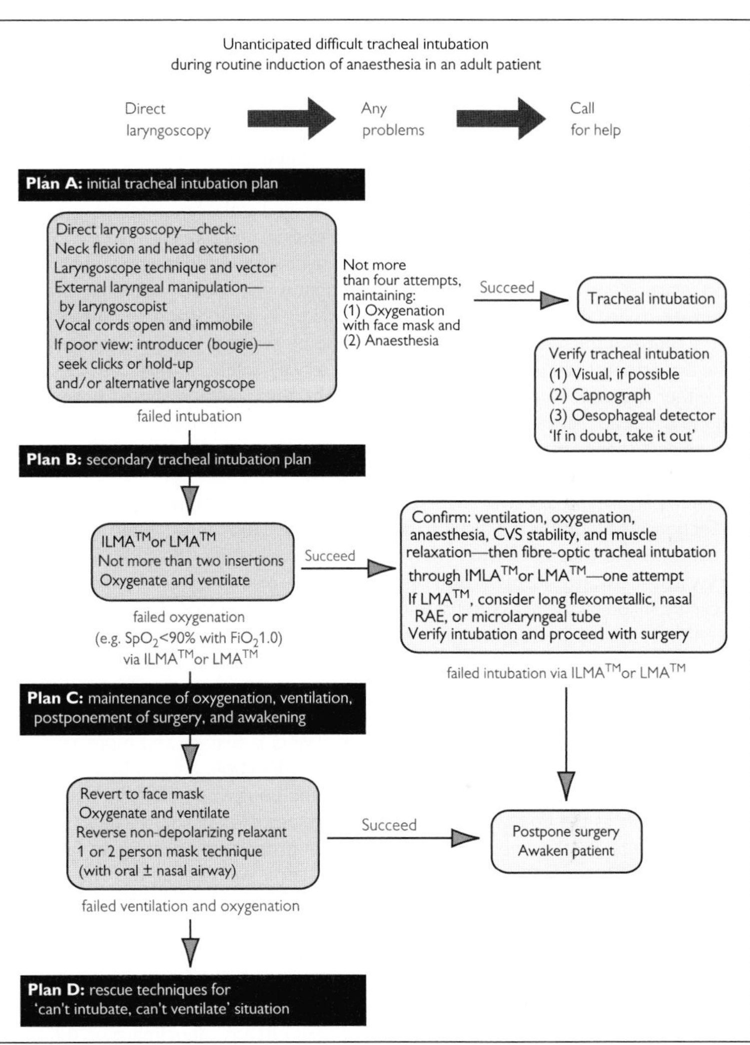

Fig 7.2 The Difficult Airway Society guidelines (2004) for the management of failed intubation during routine induction of anaesthesia.

will sequentially work through. Although most airways can be successfully managed with plan A, for every induction the anaesthetist should know what plans B, C, and D will entail.

7.2.3.1 *Plan A: initial tracheal intubation plan*

Plan A describes the anaesthetist's initial plan for intubation. This represents the first choice for airway management.

It is recognized that the airway is most easily managed at the first attempt—repeated instrumentation increases the risk of trauma, bleeding, and swelling—so every effort must be made to ensure this plan succeeds. This means optimizing patient position before starting and ensuring the correct equipment is immediately available; primarily, this means having the correct laryngoscope blade(s), in an appropriate range of sizes, and the required tracheal tube. Spares should also be available in case of device failure.

The anaesthetist should never compromise airway safety. If they are dissatisfied with either the patient position or the equipment, the induction should not proceed until the issues are resolved. Often the less senior anaesthetist may be concerned that demanding a change in position may inconvenience the surgeon, anaesthetic assistant, or patient, but safety must be the primary concern.

If, after performing direct laryngoscopy, a poor view is obtained (grade III or IV—see Section 1.3.6), or if it is difficult to pass the tracheal tube through the larynx, there are some simple measures which may improve the situation; the BURP manoeuvre (Backwards–Upwards–Rightwards–Pressure), also termed external laryngeal positioning, can be made by the anaesthetist with their free hand to move the larynx into view. Once the larynx has been positioned, the assistant can take over to maintain its position. BURP is different to cricoid pressure, in that the objective is not to occlude the oesophagus but to reposition the laryngeal inlet to improve the anaesthetist's view.

A bougie can be placed through the vocal cords prior to passing the tracheal tube. A bougie, usually made out of gum-elastic or plastic, is thinner and more rigid than a tracheal tube, making it easier to control the tip direction. Also, a bend at the tip can facilitate positioning. Correct positioning of the bougie can often be determined by feeling clicks as the tip passes over the cartilaginous rings of the trachea. 'Hold up' describes the tip of the bougie reaching the main bronchi and passing no further; if the bougie has been placed in the oesophagus then it will pass all the way into the stomach.

Once the bougie has been placed, the tracheal tube can be railroaded over the top of it. Note that it is possible to cause trauma to the airway with incautious use of a bougie.

An alternative laryngoscope (see Section 1.3.5) is the final step to be attempted in plan A. Usually this will be a device such as a McCoy laryngoscope, which has a hinged tip that can be used to elevate the epiglottis (see Fig 7.3) and often improves the laryngoscopy view by one grade. The anaesthetist should become familiar with the use of alternative laryngoscope devices, and every effort should be made to obtain training in their use in simulated or supervised clinical practice; it is not desirable to use a device for the first time in an emergency situation.

If, after not more than four attempts at intubation (using appropriate combinations of BURP, bougie, or alternative device), a tracheal tube has not been correctly sited, then the situation should be considered a 'failed intubation', and the anaesthetist should proceed to plan B.

Preoperative investigation recommendations

Adapted from NICE CG3: Preoperative Tests

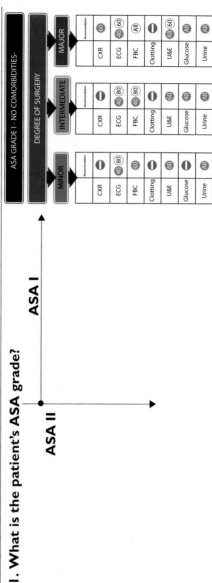

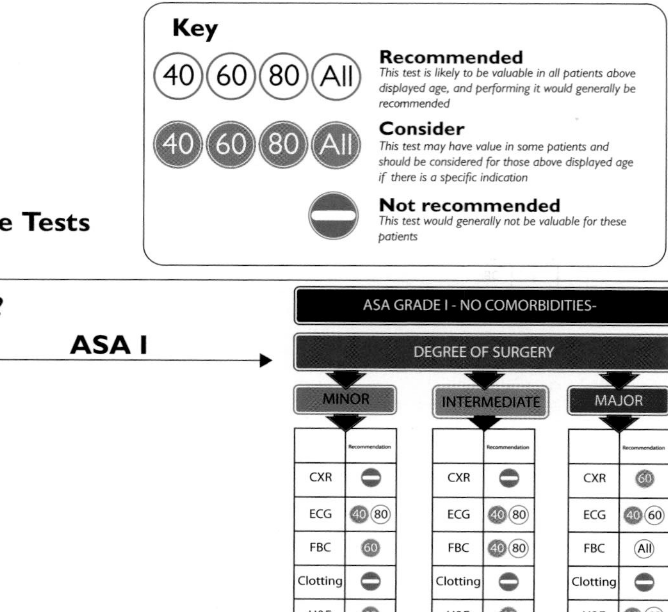

Key
40 60 80 All
Recommended
This test is likely to be valuable in all patients above displayed age, and performing it would generally be recommended
40 60 80 All
Consider
This test may have value in some patients and should be considered for those above displayed age if there is a specific indication
Not recommended
This test would generally not be valuable for these patients
1. What is the patient's ASA grade?
ASA I
ASA II
ASA GRADE I - NO COMORBIDITIES-
DEGREE OF SURGERY
MINOR
INTERMEDIATE
MAJOR

MINOR

	Recommendation
CXR	Not recommended
ECG	40 (Consider) 80 (Recommended)
FBC	60 (Consider)
Clotting	Not recommended
U&E	60 (Consider)
Glucose	Not recommended
Urine	All (Consider)

INTERMEDIATE

	Recommendation
CXR	Not recommended
ECG	40 (Consider) 80 (Recommended)
FBC	40 (Consider) 80 (Recommended)
Clotting	Not recommended
U&E	60 (Consider)
Glucose	40 (Consider)
Urine	All (Consider)

MAJOR

	Recommendation
CXR	60 (Consider)
ECG	40 (Consider) 60 (Recommended)
FBC	All (Recommended)
Clotting	Not recommended
U&E	All (Consider) 60 (Recommended)
Glucose	All (Consider)
Urine	All (Consider)

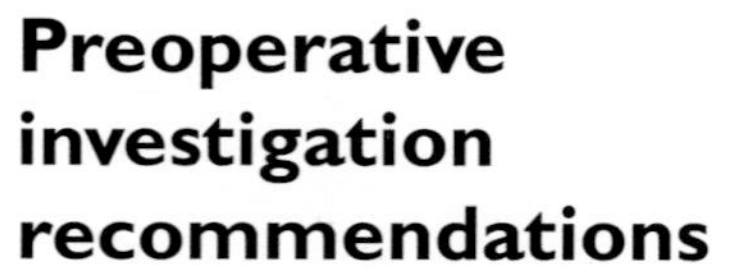

2. What are the patient's comorbidities?

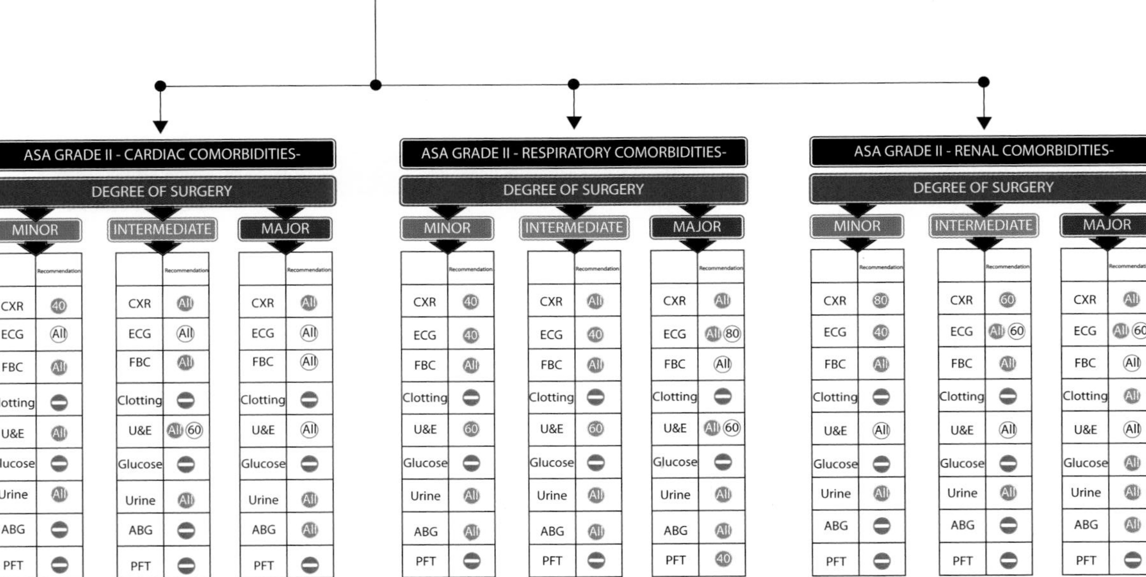

Fig 3.3 A summary of NICE guidelines *CG3: preoperative tests* (published in 2003), illustrating investigations indicated for ASA 1 and 2 patients undergoing varying degrees of surgery.

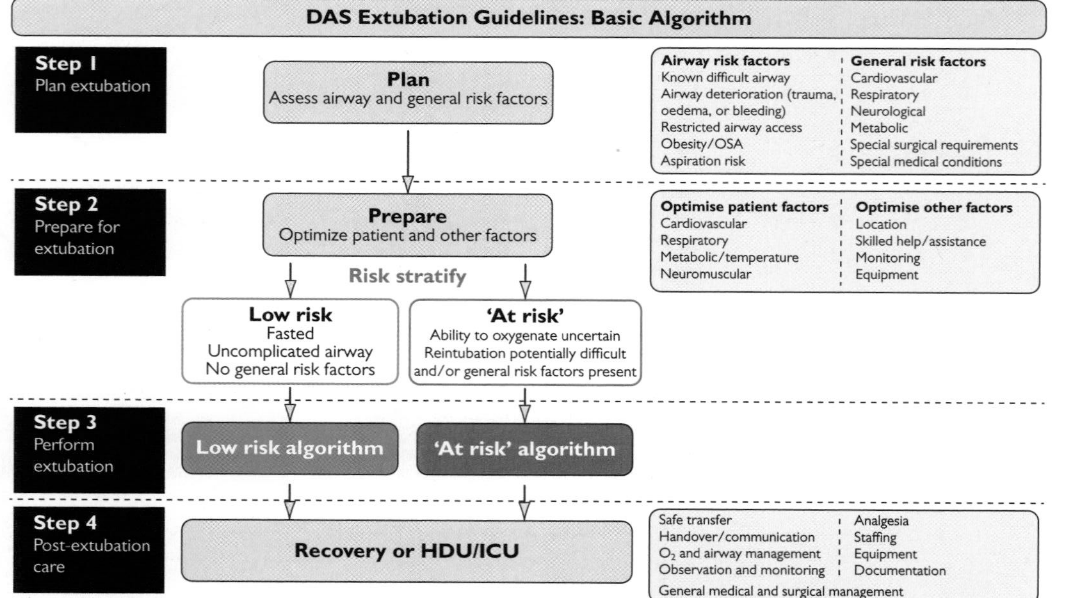

Fig 3.6a Guidelines produced by the Difficult Airway Society (2011) to help planning for extubation.

Reproduced with permission from the Difficult Airway Society.

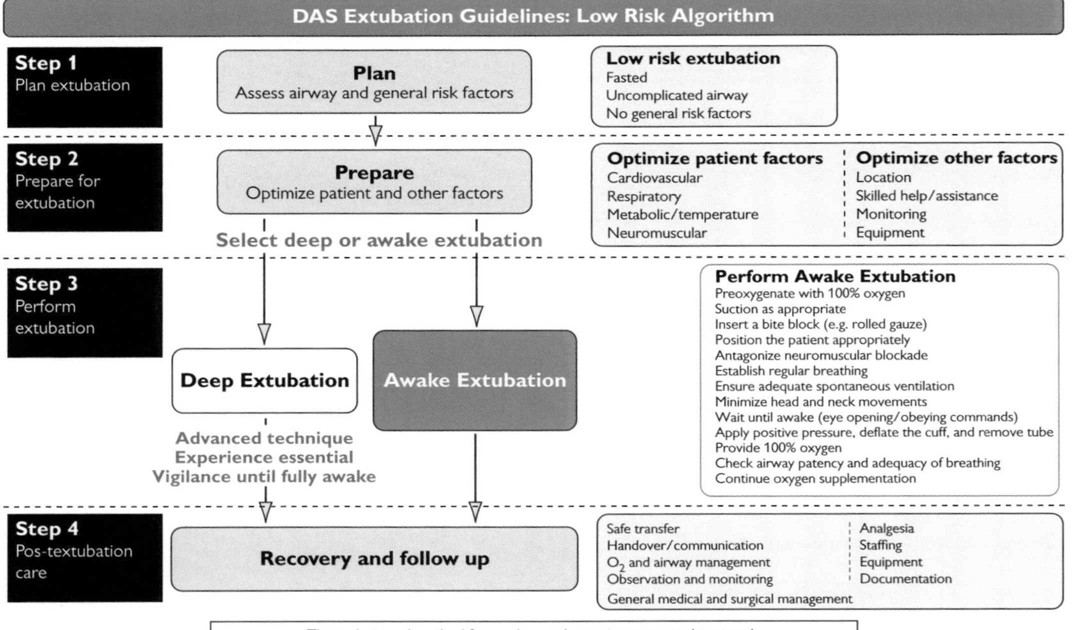

DAS Extubation Guidelines: Low Risk Algorithm
Step 1
Plan extubation
Plan
Assess airway and general risk factors
Low risk extubation
Fasted
Uncomplicated airway
No general risk factors
Step 2
Prepare for extubation
Prepare
Optimize patient and other factors
Optimize patient factors
Cardiovascular
Respiratory
Metabolic/temperature
Neuromuscular
Optimize other factors
Location
Skilled help/assistance
Monitoring
Equipment
Select deep or awake extubation
Step 3
Perform extubation
Deep Extubation
Advanced technique
Experience essential
Vigilance until fully awake
Awake Extubation
Perform Awake Extubation
Preoxygenate with 100% oxygen
Suction as appropriate
Insert a bite block (e.g. rolled gauze)
Position the patient appropriately
Antagonize neuromuscular blockade
Establish regular breathing
Ensure adequate spontaneous ventilation
Minimize head and neck movements
Wait until awake (eye opening/obeying commands)
Apply positive pressure, deflate the cuff, and remove tube
Provide 100% oxygen
Check airway patency and adequacy of breathing
Continue oxygen supplementation
Step 4
Pos-textubation care
Recovery and follow up
Safe transfer
Handover/communication
O_2 and airway management
Observation and monitoring
General medical and surgical management
Analgesia
Staffing
Equipment
Documentation
The technique described for awake extubation is a suggested approach.
Practice may vary inexperienced hands.

Fig 3.6b Guidelines produced by the Difficult Airway Society (2011) to help planning for the extubation of a low-risk airway.

Reproduced with permission from the Difficult Airway Society.

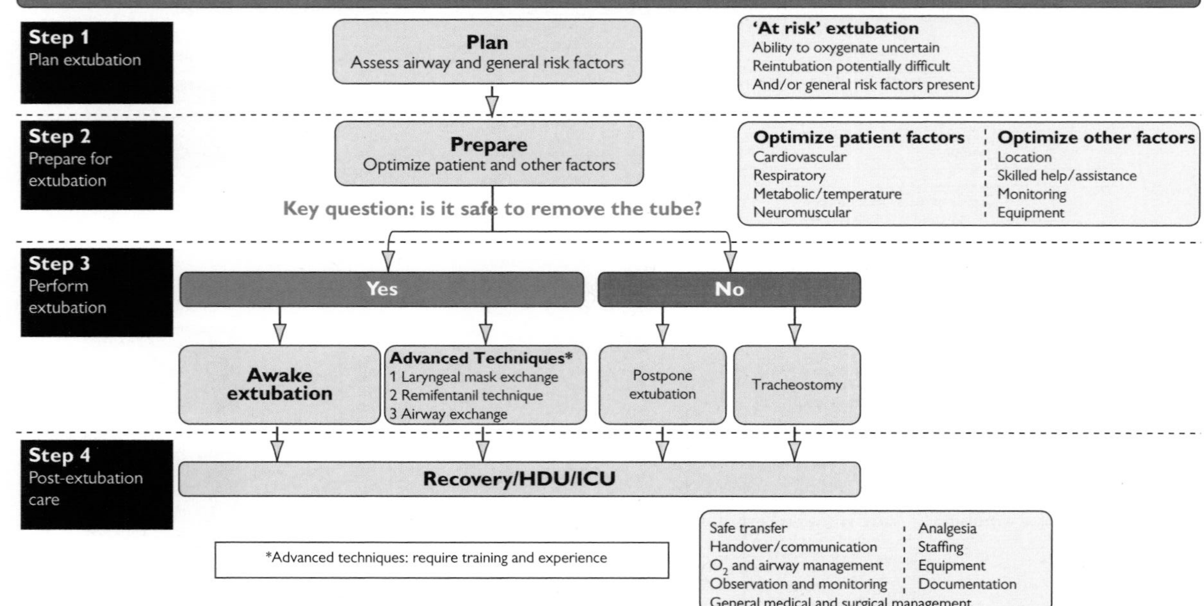

Fig 3.6c Guidelines produced by the Difficult Airway Society (2011) to help planning for the extubation of a high-risk airway.
Reproduced with permission from the Difficult Airway Society.

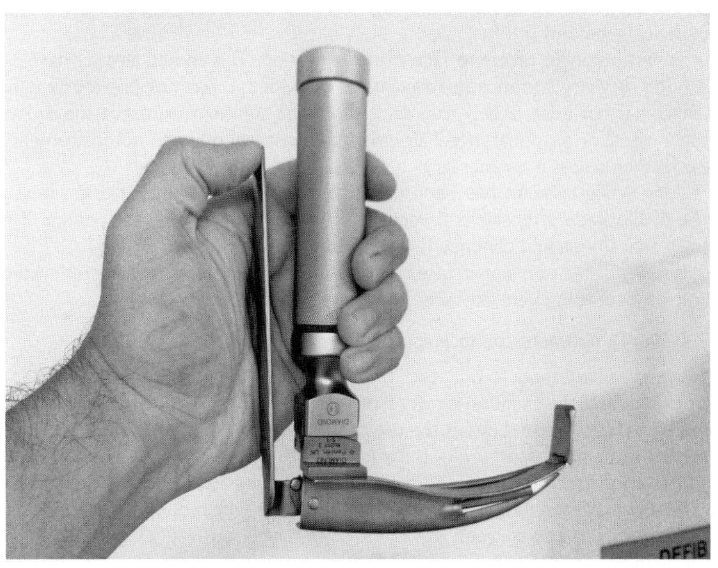

Fig 7.3 A McCoy laryngoscope. Note how depressing the handle causes the tip of the blade to hinge upwards. This can be useful to improve laryngoscopy view during difficult intubations.

7.2.3.2 *Plan B: secondary intubation plan*

If the initial plan has not been successful, the most important thing, particularly for newer anaesthetic staff, is to summon assistance immediately. The next steps may require using unfamiliar equipment, and the actions must be taken quickly and decisively. Note that a member of the scrub team is probably best placed to get help for the anaesthetist, as the anaesthetic assistant is probably the only member of the team with the airway training to help resolve the problem and should not be distracted with any other tasks at this stage.

The anaesthetist should attempt to place an intubating laryngeal mask (ILMA™)—this will permit oxygenation of the patient via the mask, while also affording a conduit through which to place a tracheal tube. Not more than two attempts should be taken to place the ILMA™.

If these measures are not successful or if, at any point, oxygen saturations fall below 90%, then oxygenation becomes the sole priority, and the anaesthetist should immediately move on to plan C.

7.2.3.3 *Plan C: maintenance of oxygenation*

If help has not already been summoned or has not arrived, it must now be called as a priority. It would be entirely appropriate to pull the emergency buzzer if help is not immediately forthcoming.

The situation at this stage is potentially very hazardous, and oxygenating the patient successfully is the only priority.

In the first instance, revert to face mask ventilation. This should already have been tried prior to giving the muscle relaxant, so, provided it was not previously difficult and there has not been airway trauma, it should be sufficient to rescue the situation. Oropharyngeal or nasopharyngeal airways may assist, although do not instrument the airway further, unless it is necessary.

If a long-acting relaxant has been used, attach a nerve stimulator and assess the degree of blockade. If possible, reverse the relaxant and wake up the patient. If not, maintain anaesthesia and continue face mask ventilation until help arrives.

If it is not possible to maintain face mask ventilation, the situation has deteriorated to a 'can't intubate–can't ventilate' scenario. This is a serious emergency.

7.2.3.4 *Plan D: airway rescue techniques*

At this stage, all attempts to maintain oxygenation are failing, and the patient is at risk of serious harm if the situation is not resolved.

Broadly, airway rescue requires the use of a 'sharp' airway—either surgical cricothyroidotomy or needle cricothyroidotomy (see Fig 7.4).

Surgical cricothyroidotomy is perhaps the 'gold standard' airway, although fewer anaesthetists may have the confidence to site one in the time required. In circumstances where a suitably trained surgeon is immediately available, e.g. in ENT or Max-Fax theatres, it would be appropriate to request their assistance.

In situations where a surgical cricothyroidotomy cannot be immediately performed, many anaesthetists would use a needle cricothyroidotomy. Kits to perform these should be available in every anaesthetic room. Although, in theory, a large IV cannula could be used, they are less suitable, because they lack the appropriate connectors to permit connection to ventilation equipment. The cannula is placed through the cricothyroid membrane, which lies between the thyroid cartilage above and the cricoid cartilage below. The cannula should be placed as close to the midline as possible. A syringe needs to be attached during placement so the anaesthetist can aspirate during the insertion; free flow of gas into the syringe suggests correct placement in the trachea.

Although larger cannula devices, such as the Rüsch QuickTrach®, can be connected to a standard 22 mm anaesthetic breathing circuit, most needle devices are of too narrow diameter to permit oxygenation without the use of a high-pressure jet ventilator (see Fig 7.5).

Jet ventilators are specialized high-pressure devices that must be connected to a dedicated oxygen supply, often a mini-Schrader valve on the anaesthetic machine itself. They deliver high-pressure/high-flow oxygen through the cannula on depression of a trigger, with a dial to control pressure. Expired gas must pass through the patient's anatomical airway, as there is no expiratory limb to a jet ventilator's pipeline.

Although ventilation (strictly, the elimination of CO_2) is poor, successful jet ventilation can maintain a patient's oxygenation for 30 min or more, which should permit sufficient time for a definitive airway to be placed.

Cricothyroidotomy is a rare event, but the techniques should be practised wherever possible. Because the equipment and methods required are seldom used, skills retention can be an issue.

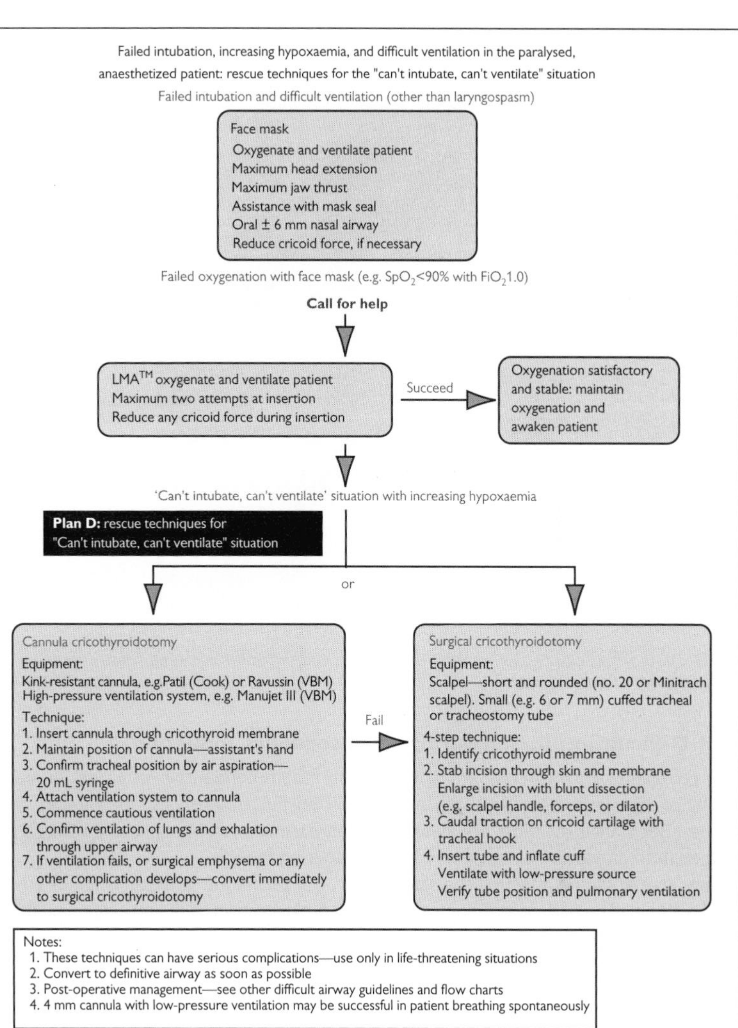

Fig 7.4 The Difficult Airway Society guidelines (2004) for the management of a 'can't intubate, can't ventilate' (CICV) scenario.

Reproduced with permission from the Difficult Airway Society.

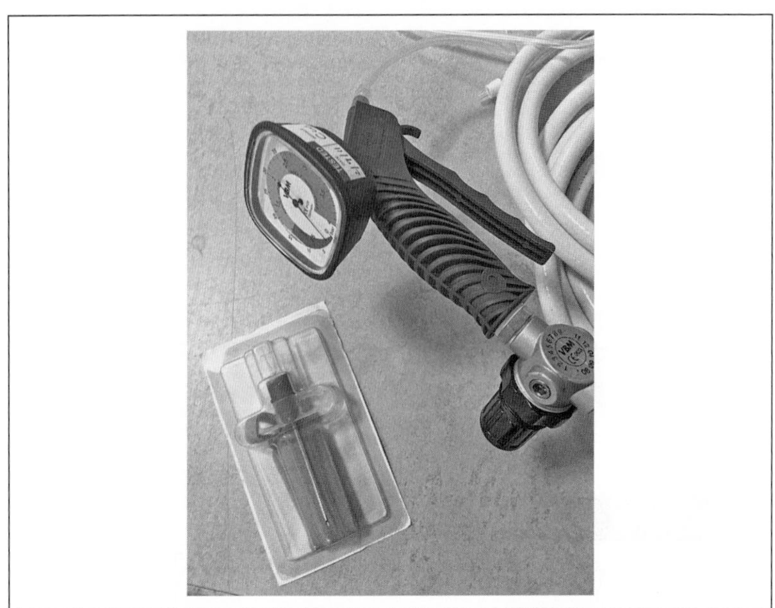

Fig 7.5 This is an example of a jet ventilator used with a needle cricothyroidotomy. These devices are usually kept on difficult airway trolleys. They take a few minutes to set up and training to use effectively.

7.2.4 **Difficult intubation during rapid sequence induction**

This guideline contains many similarities to the recommendations for failed intubation during routine induction, but there are some important differences (see Fig 7.6).

The importance of good airway assessment, careful positioning, and thorough pre-oxygenation cannot be overstated when considering the RSI.

One crucial factor affecting the safety of an RSI technique is that the ability to face mask ventilate the patient is not proved before administration of the muscle relaxant. For this reason, it is important to use short-acting muscle relaxants (e.g. suxamethonium—see Section 2.4.2.1) to ensure the patient can return to spontaneously ventilating in the shortest period if intubation fails. Administration of a second dose of suxamethonium or a long-acting muscle relaxant during an RSI is seldom recommended and should never be contemplated by the inexperienced anaesthetist.

The addition of cricoid pressure during intubation may also complicate the RSI as, if it is inexpertly applied, it may grossly distort airway findings.

7.2.4.1 *Plan A: initial tracheal intubation plan*

This is broadly similar to the initial plan at routine induction, except that reduction in cricoid pressure can be considered if the view at direct laryngoscopy is difficult. The same recommendations with regard to positioning, BURP, bougie use, and alternative laryngoscopy devices hold true.

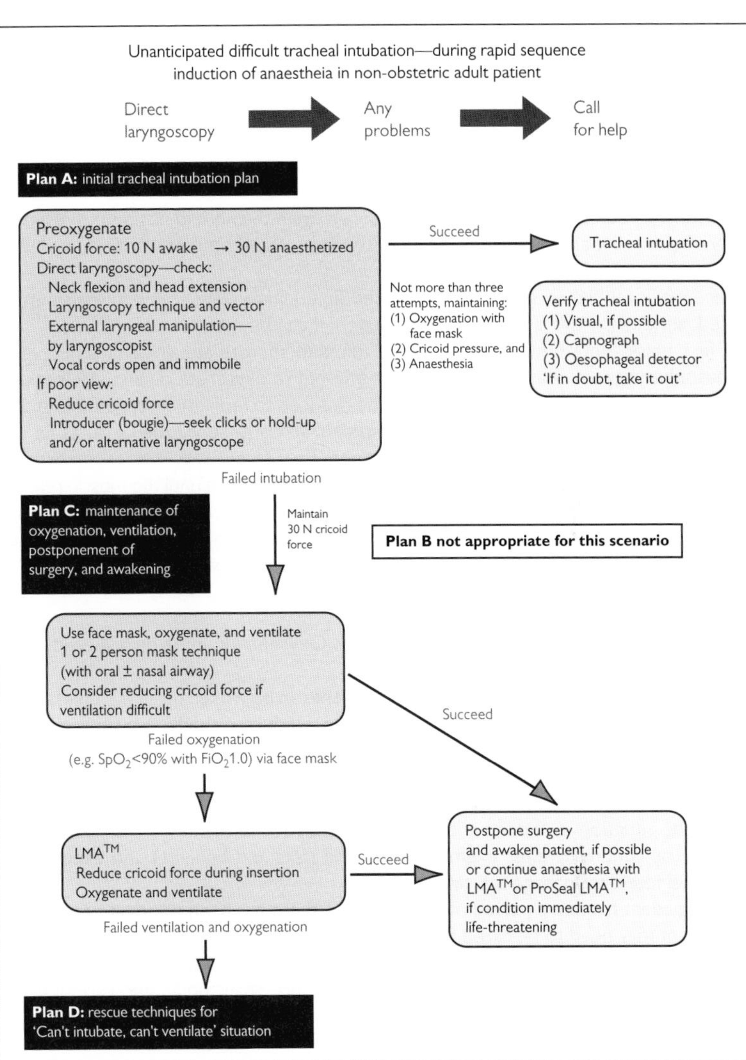

Fig 7.6 The Difficult Airway Society guidelines (2004) for the management of failed intubation during rapid sequence induction of anaesthesia.

Reproduced with permission from the Difficult Airway Society.

Only three attempts at direct laryngoscopy are permissible, reflecting the shorter time frame in which the anaesthetist must operate.

Note that there is no role for alternative intubation strategies during a rapid sequence, so in the event of failure of the initial intubation plan, the anaesthetist should omit plan B and move directly to plan C.

7.2.4.2 *Plan C: maintenance of oxygenation*

Help must be summoned immediately, although again this should not be the responsibility of either the anaesthetist or the anaesthetic assistant, both of whom must devote their attention to the patient.

Face mask ventilation should be attempted first, initially with cricoid pressure maintained, although, if this is impeding oxygenation, it can be reduced or removed.

If face mask ventilation is unsuccessful, even with appropriate airway adjuncts (oro- or nasopharyngeal airway devices), then an attempt to oxygenate via an LMA is appropriate. Again cricoid pressure may have to be reduced to facilitate insertion. Note that, in this case, there will be no attempt to pass a tracheal tube via the LMA, as its sole function is to permit oxygenation of the patient.

If oxygenation is successful, anaesthesia should be maintained until the muscle relaxant has worn off, and then the patient should be woken up. Only in truly life-threatening surgical emergencies should the procedure continue without a definitive airway in place, but this decision should be made by a senior anaesthetist and surgeon working together.

7.2.4.3 *Plan D: airway rescue techniques*

Plan D is identical to that described previously. Oxygenation must be achieved either via surgical or needle cricothyroidotomy.

Again oxygenation is maintained until the patient can be woken up safely, unless there are overwhelming surgical reasons to continue, in which case a definitive surgical airway will be required.

7.2.5 **Post-operative management and documentation**

When the situation is under control, a plan needs to be made for rescheduling the surgery (or continuing after examination of the risks and benefits) and experienced personnel found to manage the airway safely.

If the patient has had a period of hypoxia, or if there has been trauma to the airway, the patient may need to be cared for in critical care.

The anaesthetist must bear in mind that their experiences will often be crucial to informing their colleagues' management of any future anaesthetic, and careful documentation is vital. This means recording successful measures, unsuccessful techniques, and an indication of why there was difficulty.

A discussion with the patient, explaining in appropriate terms what difficulties occurred and the steps taken to resolve the situation, is essential. If the patient is aware, they can inform future anaesthetists of difficult airway problems. MedicAlert bracelets may be recommended for the patient with a difficult airway.

7.3 **Loss of capnography waveform**

The capnograph is one of the most important items of monitoring on the anaesthetic machine (see Section 1.4.4). It gives information about the presence and adequacy of ventilation, and the integrity of the breathing circuit. Its loss always requires immediate investigation. A suggested order in which to consider a loss of the capnograph waveform is presented in Fig 7.7.

7.3.1 **Airway problems**

If there has never been CO_2 present, it implies that the airway is not sited correctly, e.g. an oesophageal intubation, or that the airway is obstructed. This may be at the level of the patient, e.g. by laryngospasm, or there may be an obstruction in the breathing circuit or anaesthetic machine. If there is ever any doubt that the anaesthetic machine or breathing circuit is compromised, bag–valve–mask ventilation should be commenced to ensure adequate patient oxygenation.

7.3.2 **Disconnection**

A leak or a complete circuit disconnection is a common cause of loss of capnography. Once airway placement has been confirmed, the breathing circuit should be systematically checked, starting at the patient end and ensuring the integrity of all the connections between patient and machine. Leaks can be detected by sight, by listening for escaping gas, or by smelling a leaking anaesthetic agent.

Common sites where leaks occur:

- The connection to the airway device
- Luer lock connections on the HME filter
- Luer lock connections on the pitot tube
- The CGO
- The soda lime canister.

Note that some anaesthetic machines have an auxiliary CGO with a switch to select between primary and auxiliary outlets. Ensure that this switch is correctly positioned.

Remember that leaks can occur around the cuff of a tracheal tube or LMA.

7.3.3 **Obstruction**

If the airway or circuit becomes obstructed, the capnograph trace may be lost. Obstruction can be distinguished from a leak by squeezing the reservoir bag; with a leak, the bag will deflate and not refill fully; however, in an obstructed circuit, the bag will not deflate properly, and airway pressures will be abnormally high.

It is unusual, but not impossible, for the breathing circuit itself to be kinked. More commonly, the airway device (particularly an uncut tracheal tube) can become twisted and kinked. In cases where the patient's head must be manipulated, specially reinforced (or 'armoured') tracheal tubes are available that resist kinking.

A critical risk is a foreign body blocking the breathing circuit. Patients have died after debris (such as the cap from an IV line) blocked anaesthetic circuits (see Figs 7.8a and 7.8b). The Department of Health produced guidelines in 2004 on the safe handling of circuits to minimize these risks.

In the event of obstruction, check the circuit. If a cause cannot be found, the circuit must be replaced. It is usually best to switch to a self-inflating bag as a temporary measure. Remember that obstructions can occur distal to the HME filter, so, if the patient's

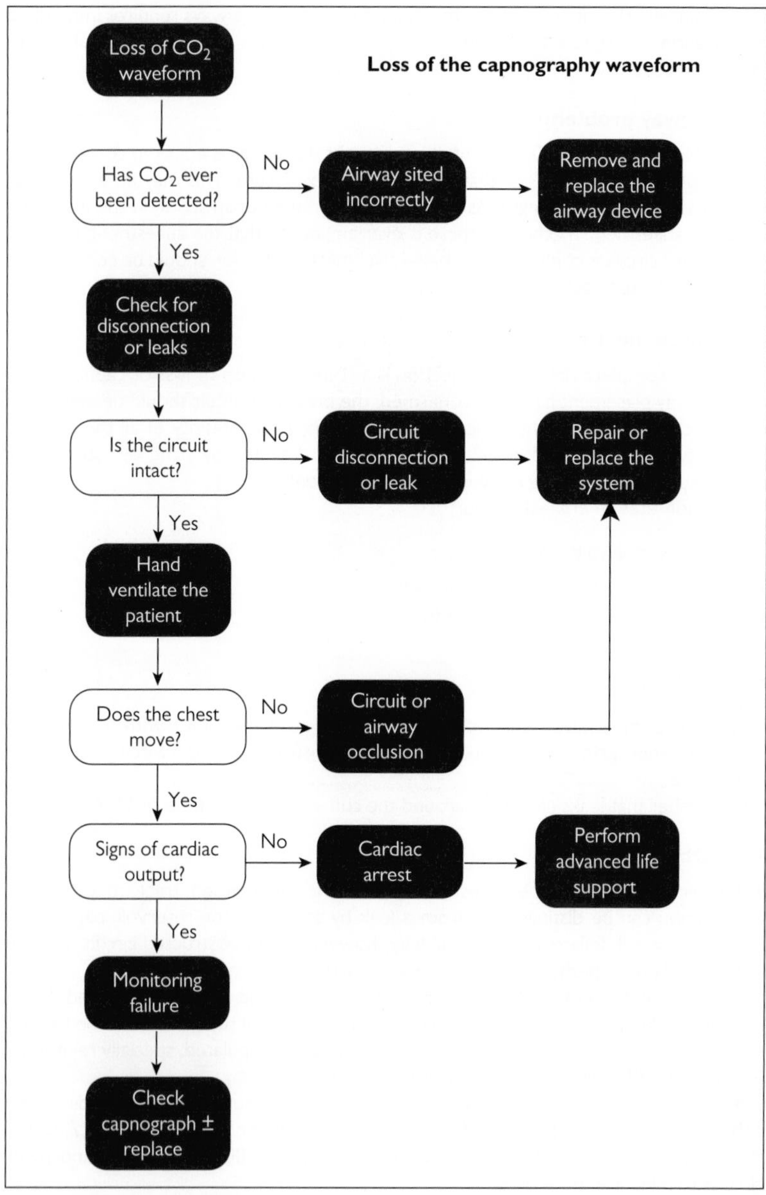

Fig 7.7 A suggested flow chart for the investigation of a loss of capnography waveform during general anaesthesia.

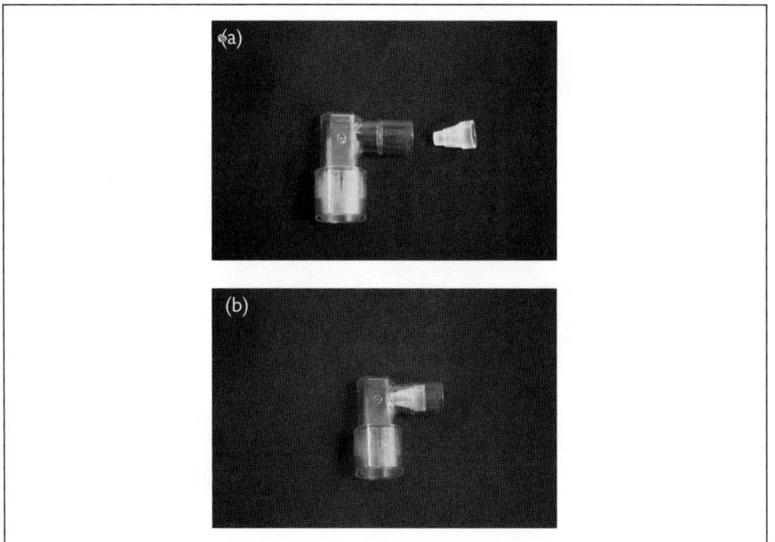

Figs 7.8a and b This illustrates how an IV line cap can easily block a breathing circuit. Great care must be taken to ensure that foreign bodies cannot contaminate the anaesthetic systems.

lungs still cannot be ventilated, consider replacing the filter, the angle-piece, and catheter mount, and even the airway itself.

7.3.4 **Cardiac arrest**

If the airway is patent and there are no leaks within the circuit, then it implies that the patient is either no longer generating CO_2 or not delivering that CO_2 to the lungs.

A central pulse should be checked immediately, and, if appropriate, life support must be commenced (see Section 7.9).

7.3.5 **Monitoring failure**

Failure of monitoring equipment is a diagnosis of exclusion. It is rare, and only if all other causes have been considered and eliminated would this be considered; the monitor should be immediately replaced. It is not appropriate to continue a case without capnography.

7.4 High airway pressures

High airway pressures put the patient at risk of barotrauma and pneumothorax. Problems can arise through faults in monitoring equipment, problems with the breathing circuit or airway device, or because the patient has developed respiratory pathology. A suggested order in which to consider high airway pressure is presented in Fig 7.9.

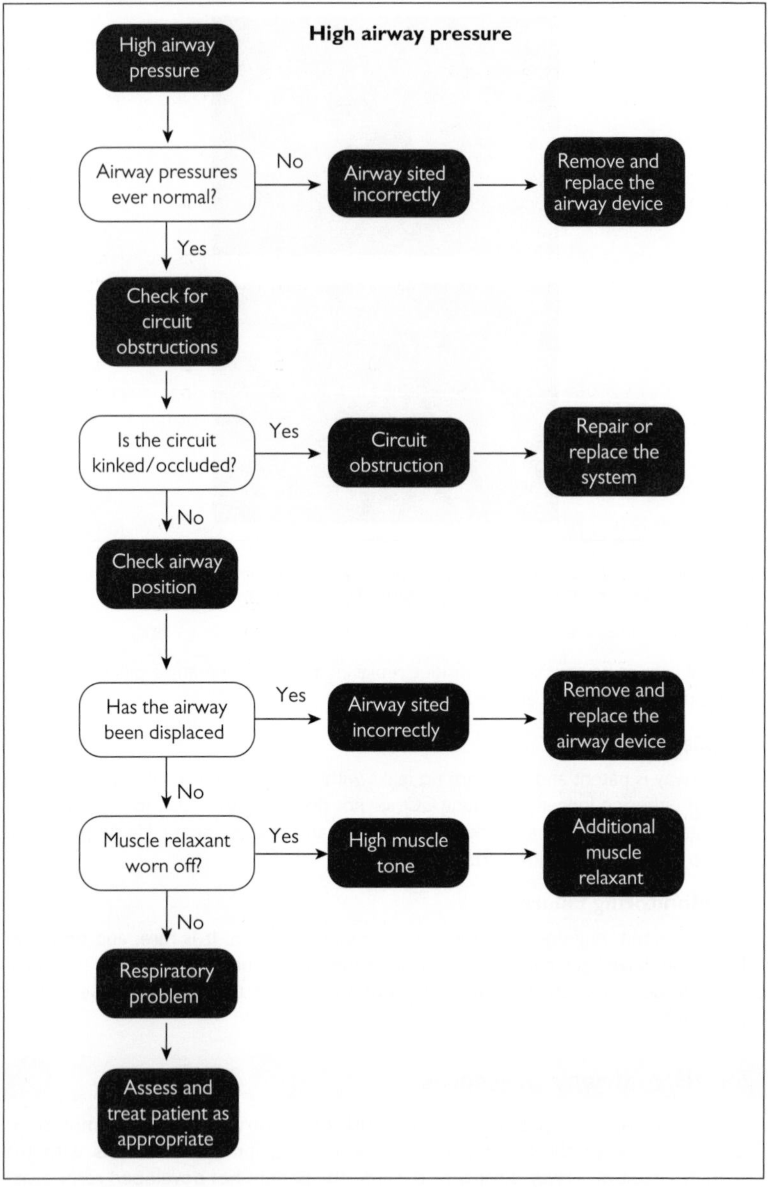

Fig 7.9 A suggested flow chart for the investigation of high airway pressures during general anaesthesia.

7.4.1 **Airway problems**

If airway pressures have always been high, it is likely that the airway is not correctly sited. In the case of a laryngeal mask, this may represent the cuff not sitting correctly in the pharynx or the epiglottis partially obstructing the airway. In these cases, the LMA will need to be removed and replaced.

In the case of a tracheal tube, endobronchial intubation should be excluded. Check the depth markings on the tube; in an average-sized adult, the tube should not be inserted beyond 24 cm at the teeth. Withdrawing the tube may be all that is required to correct the airway pressures.

If airway pressures remain high, in spite of manipulating the airway, consider obstruction as a possible cause, and replace the airway with a checked, brand-new device.

7.4.2 **Obstruction**

A new rise in airway pressure means the circuit should be checked for obstructions or kinking. The airway device should be included in this check. Start from the patient end, and work backwards towards the anaesthetic machine. If using a circle system, check that the unidirectional valves are functioning correctly.

7.4.3 **Airway displacement**

Another source of airway obstruction is displacement of the airway. An airway can be accidentally withdrawn, causing leak or complete loss, but it is also possible for movement to push a tracheal tube in further, which may result in ventilating only one lung (endobronchial intubation). Laryngeal masks can also become displaced.

The airway should be inspected and replaced, as appropriate. If the airway must be manipulated during a case, make sure the anaesthetic assistant is present, and pre-oxygenate the patient beforehand, if possible. This will maximize the time available to correct the problem.

7.4.4 **Muscle relaxation**

Muscle relaxants reduce thoracic wall tone, which reduces airway pressures. As the drug wears off and tone returns, a gradual increase in airway pressures is detectable. This is only usually a significant problem if the patient is obese or has a particularly muscular chest wall.

Once the neuromuscular blockade has worn off entirely, sudden surgical or airway stimulus can cause the patient to cough. This will result in sudden, large spikes in airway pressure.

A peripheral nerve stimulator should be used to check the state of neuromuscular blockade and an appropriate relaxant dose given, if required.

7.4.5 **Reduced pulmonary compliance**

If the circuit is intact and an appropriate level of muscle relaxation has been achieved, but airway pressures remain high, the anaesthetist should consider intrinsic lung pathologies.

Many acute conditions can reduce pulmonary compliance intraoperatively and cause increases in airway pressure:

- **Bronchoconstriction:** auscultate the chest, listening for expiratory wheeze. Deepening volatile anaesthesia (ideally with sevoflurane, as it is less irritant than isoflurane) can reduce bronchoconstriction due to bronchodilator effects, but β-agonist therapy may be required. It is possible to deliver inhaled or nebulized drugs into an anaesthetic circuit, but this requires a specialized breathing circuit adaptor, which may not be immediately available in all theatres. IV salbutamol (250 micrograms by slow IV injection) can also be used, while ketamine has bronchodilator properties, making it a useful second-line agent

- **Mucus plugging:** mucus plugs in a large bronchus can cause raised airway pressures. Signs might include coarse inspiratory and expiratory noises or reduced breath sounds in the affected zone. Passing a suction catheter down the airway can remove such plugs
- **Pulmonary oedema:** increased tissue interstitial pressures, caused by pulmonary oedema, stiffens the lung, raising airway pressures. Signs include fine inspiratory crepitations and raised venous pressures. Definitive treatment would be diuretic therapy, but oxygenation can be improved by increasing positive end-expiratory pressure (PEEP), which helps to push fluid from the alveoli, although at the expense of raising airway pressures further
- **Pneumothorax:** pneumothorax developing during anaesthesia requires prompt intervention as there is high risk of the pneumothorax tensioning, especially in ventilated patients. Diagnosis is made by detecting absent or reduced breath sounds, along with hyperresonance on the affected side. Tracheal deviation is a very late sign of a tension pneumothorax. Needle decompression, using a large-gauge IV cannula in the second intercostal space and mid-clavicular line, will give immediate relief, but an intercostal chest drain is the definitive treatment
- **Surgery:** surgical factors can impact on airway pressures, most obviously as the abdomen is inflated during laparoscopic surgery. Raised intra-abdominal pressures are transmitted into the chest and can make ventilation difficult, especially if the patient is placed in a head-down position. Reducing the I:E ratio and switching from volume-controlled to pressure-controlled ventilation may reduce pressures to acceptable levels. If this is not sufficient, it is necessary to ask the surgeons to reduce the intra-abdominal pressure and/or place the patient in a less steep head-down position.

7.5 Airway problems at extubation

Airway problems are most commonly thought of in regard to induction of general anaesthesia, but it is important to remember that extubation at the end of surgery carries as many risks. It can even be more hazardous after procedures in or around the airway. The anaesthetist must remain vigilant and prepared for unanticipated problems until the patient is fully awake (see Box 7.2). Guidelines exist for the planning of extubation (see Section 3.4.3).

Box 7.2 Learning point

Remember: **never take out an airway that you are not prepared to put back**.

7.5.1 **Extubation of the low-risk airway**

Prior to extubation, steps must be taken to prepare the patient. First, the anaesthetist must check that the patient is suitable for extubation by ensuring normothermia, correcting acidosis, and confirming cardiovascular stability.

Determine the plan for extubation. Patients who are fasted, are not an aspiration risk, and who have not had an airway-related procedure may be suitable for a deep extubation. Deep extubation should be performed only under the supervision of experienced anaesthetists and where there is no risk of aspiration.

If there is any risk of airway soiling, the patient must be extubated awake.

7.5.1.1 *Awake extubation*

Awake extubation is usually the safest extubation strategy and is generally the preferred option for less experienced anaesthetists. The patient should be preoxygenated prior to extubation. Use a nerve stimulator to check that there is no residual neuromuscular blockade, and reverse as appropriate. Discontinue the anaesthetic agent, and suction the airway carefully to remove any secretions. Monitoring should be continued until the tube has been removed and the patient is stable.

Position the patient in a semi-supine position where you can easily reach both the airway and the anaesthetic machine. Mechanical ventilation can be continued until the patient's respiratory effort takes over. Make sure the anaesthetic assistant is present and that you have prepared equipment to reintubate, if necessary. Also ensure extra doses of propofol and suxamethonium are available in the event of laryngospasm (see Section 7.5.3).

When the patient eye-opens to command or makes a purposeful movement towards the tracheal tube, the cuff can be deflated and the tube removed.

After extubation, connect a face mask to the anaesthetic circuit, and place the mask over the patient's mouth and nose. Watch for bag movements and capnography to ensure the adequacy of ventilation. Airway manoeuvres may be needed to maintain the airway initially.

Once adequate respiratory effort has been confirmed, replace the anaesthetic face mask with a Hudson mask connected to a high-flow oxygen supply.

The patient can be taken to the recovery room when the anaesthetist is satisfied that their airway is patent and that their respiratory effort is adequate. Although recovery staff can perform basic airway manoeuvres, a patient should not leave theatre if there is doubt about the airway.

7.5.1.2 *Deep extubation*

Deep extubation has advantages under certain circumstances, as there is a lower incidence of coughing which may be an advantage in some specialist surgical circumstances.

The technique is performed only under the supervision of experienced anaesthetists and where there is no risk of airway soiling.

The patient is preoxygenated and positioned as for an awake extubation, except the anaesthetic agent is not withdrawn until after the tube has been removed. Again, monitoring must be continued throughout the extubation process.

While the patient is still anaesthetized, check that there is no ongoing neuromuscular blockade. Mechanical ventilation is then discontinued. Once the patient has stable spontaneous respiratory effort, and after full preoxygenation, the airway must be carefully suctioned. The tracheal tube cuff can be deflated, but without withdrawing the tube. Watch the patient's respiratory effort for a further few minutes, and, if respirations continue to be stable, the tube can be removed. Revert to an anaesthetic face mask, maintain the airway, and ensure that spontaneous respiratory effort continues. Only then should the anaesthetic agent be withdrawn and the patient permitted to wake. An oropharyngeal airway to assist with airway maintenance is useful.

The patient will be slower to wake, as the anaesthetic agent is withdrawn later in the process. It is therefore vital that the anaesthetist monitors the patient prior to transfer until such time as the patient can maintain their own airway.

It is dangerous to perform an extubation in light planes of anaesthesia, so, if the anaesthetic agent has been discontinued prior to extubation, proceed to an awake extubation.

7.5.2 **Extubation of the high-risk airway**

The most commonly encountered 'at-risk' airway is in the non-fasted patient after emergency surgery. Under these circumstances, the only safe extubation strategy is fully awake.

The technique is similar to that described previously, except that the non-fasted patient is usually best extubated in the left lateral position. Extubation should only occur on a bed or trolley that can rapidly be tipped into a head-down position. This ensures that, should reflux of gastric contents occur, material is carried into the mouth and not into the larynx.

Where patients have a difficult airway—that is, they are a difficult intubation or are difficult to face mask ventilate—extubation should only occur under the direct supervision of a senior anaesthetist, as this carries significant risks.

In a proportion of patients extubation is not appropriate, and they must be electively ventilated in an intensive care environment until the airway difficulty has resolved.

If there is ever any doubt about the safety of extubation, consult with a senior colleague before attempting to proceed.

7.5.3 **Laryngospasm**

Laryngospasm on extubation can cause rapid and significant hypoxia.

Although it can occur at any time, it is more common after airway surgery, in non-fasted patients, in children, or after significant vagal stimulus.

It is recognized by inspiratory stridor, see-saw abdominal and chest movements, or complete airway obstruction.

If the patient has been inadequately preoxygenated prior to extubation, oxygen saturations will fall rapidly. After proper preoxygenation, there will be a period of a few minutes in which to correct the problem.

The first step is to recognize the problem. Many episodes of laryngospasm will respond simply to PEEP. This can be achieved by closing the APL valve to 10–20 cmH_2O.

If this is not rapidly successful, deepening anaesthesia will be required. This is best achieved with propofol, as this agent also suppresses airway reflexes. A dose of 0.5–1 mg/kg may be required. Assistance from an anaesthetic colleague should be sought urgently.

If deepening anaesthesia is not successful, and particularly if the patient is desaturating, suxamethonium (0.25 mg/kg) will be required. This dose should cause laryngeal relaxation without generalized paralysis. If laryngospasm progresses to this stage, it would be appropriate to sound the emergency buzzer.

The patient should be monitored in theatre until fully awake, as laryngospasm can recur.

7.6 Suxamethonium apnoea

Suxamethonium apnoea is an inherited condition where the patient lacks the plasma cholinesterase enzymes that metabolize the depolarizing neuromuscular-blocking agent suxamethonium (see Section 2.4.2.1), prolonging its action beyond the 5–8 min normally seen.

The severity of suxamethonium apnoea depends on the genotype that the patient has; up to 1:25 people possess a heterozygous-atypical genotype that mildly prolongs the action of suxamethonium (by up to 10–12 min). In contrast, patients with a homozygous-silent genotype may remain paralysed for several hours after suxamethonium.

Certain acquired conditions may give clinical pictures similar to suxamethonium apnoea. Pregnancy, liver disease, renal failure, and certain drugs may all affect plasma cholinesterase activity. Acquired deficiencies of cholinesterase do not usually prolong suxamethonium activity by more than a few minutes.

Suxamethonium apnoea is not an emergency provided it is recognized before waking the patient up. After an induction in which suxamethonium has been used, it is good practice not to give a non-depolarizing agent until there are signs that the suxamethonium has worn off, either by checking with a nerve stimulator or by the patient showing signs of restoration of neuromuscular transmission. In cases where there is no return of neuromuscular function by the end of the case, it is usually a matter of prolonging anaesthesia and continuing to mechanically ventilate the patient until the drug effect has worn off. In theory, fresh frozen plasma, which contains plasma cholinesterase, could be used as an antidote.

If a patient is suspected of having suxamethonium apnoea, it is important to discuss this with them afterwards and, if the patient is willing, to arrange for them and their family to be tested. The patient should also be told they need to warn future anaesthetists.

Atracurium, rocuronium, and vecuronium (see Section 2.4.1) can all be used safely in patients with suxamethonium apnoea, and no dose adjustment is required. There is however, one non-depolarizing agent (mivacurium) that is metabolized by the same plasma cholinesterases as suxamethonium, so suxamethonium apnoea patients should not receive this drug.

7.7 Anaphylaxis

Anaphylaxis is a life-threatening condition that requires prompt recognition to treat effectively. Many anaesthetic agents are potential triggers; muscle relaxants, antibiotics, and colloids are particularly common triggers of in-theatre anaphylaxis.

Anaphylaxis may also be encountered by the anaesthetist in other departments when they are called to provide airway assistance.

In common with all critically ill patients, initial assessment should take the 'A to E' approach. Patients with anaphylaxis are at risk from airway oedema, and consideration should be given to early intubation if there are signs of airway involvement. Cardiovascular collapse is very common. Only half of patients will display the characteristic rash, and the diagnosis should be considered in any patient with significant and intractable hypotension.

Management guidelines published by the Resuscitation Council (UK) are reproduced in Fig 7.10.

7.7.1 **First-line treatment**

Immediate management consists of removing the trigger agent, e.g. by discontinuing an antibiotic infusion, and putting the patient on high-flow oxygen. If there are signs of airway obstruction, the patient may need intubation quickly.

First-line therapy is with adrenaline (see Section 2.5.1.3). In the ward environment, adrenaline should always be given IM. The correct dose is 500 micrograms (0.5 mL of a 1:1000 solution). This dose can be repeated after 5 min, if required. The AAGBI recommends IV therapy be considered for patients in theatre, but this is reserved for anaesthetists with sufficient experience of handling and diluting adrenaline, as the consequences of an error can be significant.

Anaphylaxis patients are likely to need fluid resuscitation. Crystalloid solutions, such as Hartmann's or 0.9% saline, are best, as colloids are potential triggers of anaphylaxis themselves. Large fluid volumes may be necessary.

7.7.2 **Second-line management**

When time permits, second-line agents should be administered:

- Hydrocortisone 200 mg IV
- Chlorphenamine 10–20 mg IV.

Blood samples should be taken for tryptase, an enzyme released by mast cell degranulation. A sample should be taken as close to the event as possible, and repeat samples taken at 1–2 h and 24 h. It is the responsibility of the anaesthetist to organize sampling for cases that have occurred in theatre.

The event should be carefully documented and the patient informed. All patients should be referred to a specialist allergy service for immunology follow-up.

7.8 **Local anaesthetic toxicity**

7.8.1 **Presenting features of local anaesthetic toxicity**

LA toxicity is a potentially fatal complication of any LA, but with care it is preventable.

LA toxicity develops after either (1) exceeding the maximum safe dose for the drug or (2) an accidental IV injection.

LA drugs act to block sodium ion channels, which are widespread throughout all excitable tissues in the body. The effects of toxic doses of LA are therefore varied, but classically LA toxicity is described as presenting initially with circumoral numbness,

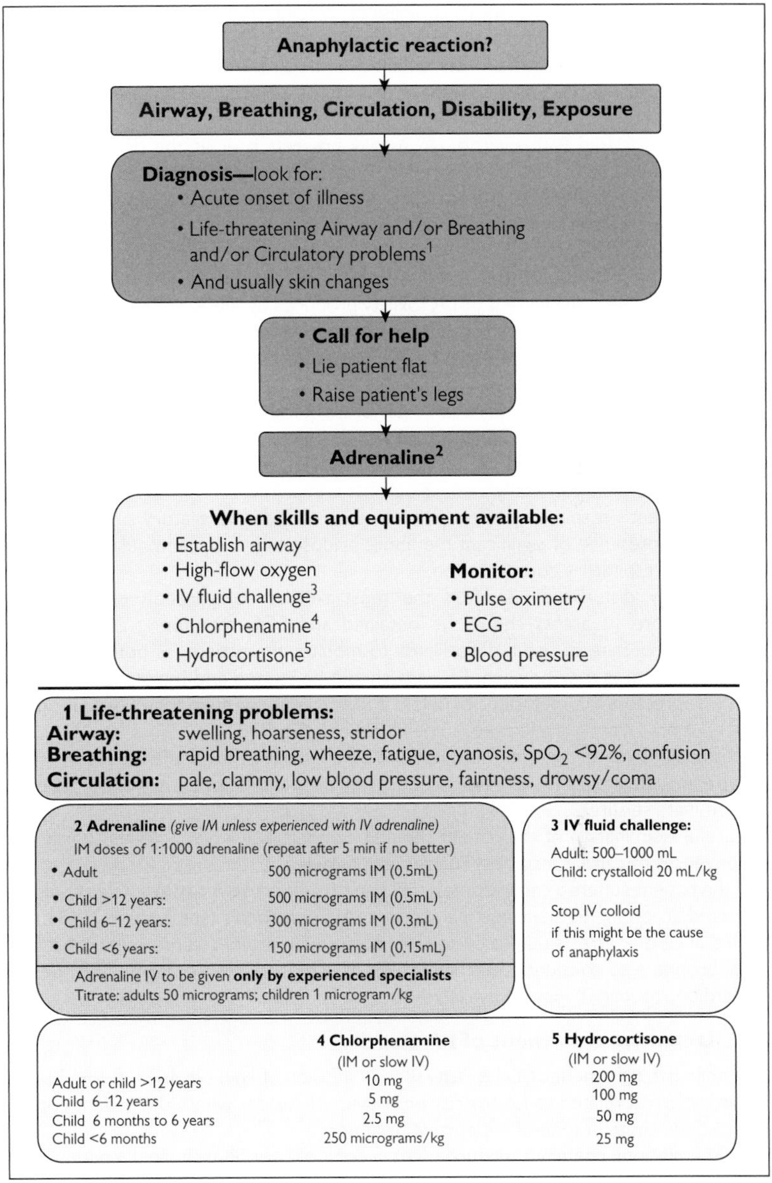

Anaphylactic reaction?

↓

Airway, Breathing, Circulation, Disability, Exposure

↓

Diagnosis—look for:
- Acute onset of illness
- Life-threatening Airway and/or Breathing and/or Circulatory problems[1]
- And usually skin changes

↓

- **Call for help**
- Lie patient flat
- Raise patient's legs

↓

Adrenaline[2]

↓

When skills and equipment available:
- Establish airway
- High-flow oxygen
- IV fluid challenge[3]
- Chlorphenamine[4]
- Hydrocortisone[5]

Monitor:
- Pulse oximetry
- ECG
- Blood pressure

---

1 Life-threatening problems:

Airway: swelling, hoarseness, stridor
Breathing: rapid breathing, wheeze, fatigue, cyanosis, SpO_2 <92%, confusion
Circulation: pale, clammy, low blood pressure, faintness, drowsy/coma

2 Adrenaline *(give IM unless experienced with IV adrenaline)*

IM doses of 1:1000 adrenaline (repeat after 5 min if no better)

• Adult	500 micrograms IM (0.5mL)
• Child >12 years:	500 micrograms IM (0.5mL)
• Child 6–12 years:	300 micrograms IM (0.3mL)
• Child <6 years:	150 micrograms IM (0.15mL)

Adrenaline IV to be given **only by experienced specialists**
Titrate: adults 50 micrograms; children 1 microgram/kg

3 IV fluid challenge:

Adult: 500–1000 mL
Child: crystalloid 20 mL/kg

Stop IV colloid if this might be the cause of anaphylaxis

	4 Chlorphenamine (IM or slow IV)	**5 Hydrocortisone** (IM or slow IV)
Adult or child >12 years	10 mg	200 mg
Child 6–12 years	5 mg	100 mg
Child 6 months to 6 years	2.5 mg	50 mg
Child <6 months	250 micrograms/kg	25 mg

Fig 7.10 Guidelines for the management of anaphylaxis (2010).

Reproduced with the kind permission of the Resuscitation Council (UK).

followed by altered consciousness, convulsions, respiratory failure, and cardiovascular collapse. Cardiac arrest may be the presenting feature.

LA toxicity can occur immediately on injection of an LA drug. This is usually a sign of intravascular injection and is perhaps most likely to occur when injecting into an epidural catheter or during peripheral nerve blocks.

Toxicity associated with overdosage usually presents later as the drug takes time to be absorbed. The speed of absorption varies, depending on the site of injection, generally being absorbed faster from vascular sites, such as the intrapleural space, than poorly perfused areas around peripheral nerves.

7.8.2 **Initial management of LA toxicity**

Guidelines for the management of LA toxicity produced by the AAGBI are reproduced in Figs 7.11a and 7.11b. After recognizing LA toxicity, the most important thing is to stop injecting the drug. If the patient is connected to a pump, e.g. giving an epidural infusion, this should be stopped and disconnected.

Call for help early, as the patient can deteriorate quickly. Initial management steps are supportive, following the ABCDE pattern.

Give high-flow oxygen, and support the airway. The airway may need to be secured with a tracheal tube, especially if consciousness is impaired.

If the patient's respiratory effort is inadequate consider ventilatory support, especially in the presence of significant metabolic acidosis where hyperventilation may be required as respiratory compensation.

Circulatory disturbance is often the most serious complication of LA toxicity. Large-bore IV access should be obtained and ECG monitoring connected. It may be appropriate to use a defibrillator to monitor the patient, as both tachy- and brady-arrhythmias may be seen. IV fluids should be started and hypotension treated with vasopressors like metaraminol (avoid if bradycardic) or ephedrine (avoid if tachycardic). If bradycardia is a feature, atropine may be required.

Convulsions can occur, and these need to be controlled using benzodiazepines. If in theatre and the airway is secure, small doses of thiopentone or propofol can be used to terminate seizures.

Careful examination of the patient should be undertaken when possible to rule out other causes of cardiac instability such as anaphylaxis.

If the patient suffers a cardiac arrest, in spite of supportive measures, this should be managed according to advanced life support (ALS) protocols (see Section 7.9.1), but note that cardiac arrests due to LA toxicity may require prolonged resuscitation. It may be appropriate to consider a mechanical cardiopulmonary resuscitation (CPR) device or cardiopulmonary bypass, if available.

7.8.3 **Definitive treatment of LA toxicity**

The definitive treatment of LA toxicity is an IV infusion of lipid emulsion. It is indicated in cardiac arrest related to LA toxicity or in cases of toxicity where the patient continues to deteriorate in spite of supportive treatment.

Lipid emulsions contain a mixture of soya bean oil, egg phospholipid, and glycerin. Although lipid emulsions form the base of parenteral nutrition and drugs like propofol, neither are suitable alternatives.

AAGBI safety guideline

Management of severe local anaesthetic toxicity

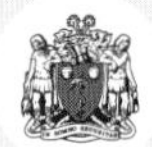

1 Recognition	**Signs of severe toxicity:** • Sudden alteration in mental status, severe agitation, or loss of consciousness, with or without tonic-clonic convulsions • Cardiovascular collapse: sinus bradycardia, conduction blocks, asystole, and ventricular tachyarrhythmias may all occur • Local anaesthetic (LA) toxicity may occur some time after an initial injection
2 Immediate management	• Stop injecting the LA • Call for help • Maintain the airway and, if necessary, secure it with a tracheal tube • Give 100% oxygen and ensure adequate lung ventilation (hyperventilation may help by increasing plasma pH in the presence of metabolic acidosis) • Confirm or establish intravenous access • Control seizures: give a benzodiazepine, thiopental, or propofol in small incremental doses • Assess cardiovascular status throughout • Consider drawing blood for analysis, but do not delay definitive treatment to do this
3 Treatment	**IN CIRCULATORY ARREST** • Start cardiopulmonary resuscitation (CPR) using standard protocols • Manage arrhythmias using the same protocols, recognizing that arrhythmias may be very refractory to treatment • Consider the use of cardiopulmonary bypass if available **GIVE INTRAVENOUS LIPID EMULSION** (following the regimen overleaf) • Continue CPR throughout treatment with lipid emulsion • Recovery from LA-induced cardiac arrest may take >1 h • Propofol is not a suitable substitute for lipid emulsion • Lidocaine should not be used as an anti-arrhythmic therapy **WITHOUT CIRCULATORY ARREST** Use conventional therapies to treat: • Hypotension • Bradycardia • Tachyarrhythmia **CONSIDER INTRAVENOUS LIPID EMULSION** (following the regimen overleaf) • Propofol is not a suitable substitute for lipid emulsion • Lidocaine should not be used as an anti-arrhythmic therapy
4 Follow-up	• Arrange safe transfer to a clinical area with appropriate equipment and suitable staff until sustained recovery is achieved • Exclude pancreatitis by regular clinical review, including daily amylase or lipase assays for 2 days • Report cases as follows: in the UK to the National Patient Safety Agency (**http://www.npsa.nhs.uk**) in the Republic of Ireland to the Irish Medicines Board (via **http://www.imb.ie**) If lipid has been given, please also report its use to the international registry at **http://www.lipidregistry.org** Details may also be posted at **http://www.lipidrescue.org**

Your nearest bag of lipid emulsion is kept. ....

This guideline is not a standard of medical care. The ultimate judgement with regard to a particular clinical procedure or treatment plan must be made by the clinician in the light of the clinical data presented and the diagnostic and treatment options available.

Fig 7.11a, b Guidelines for the management of LA toxicity (2010).
Reproduced with the kind permission of the Association of Anaesthetists of Great Britain and Ireland.

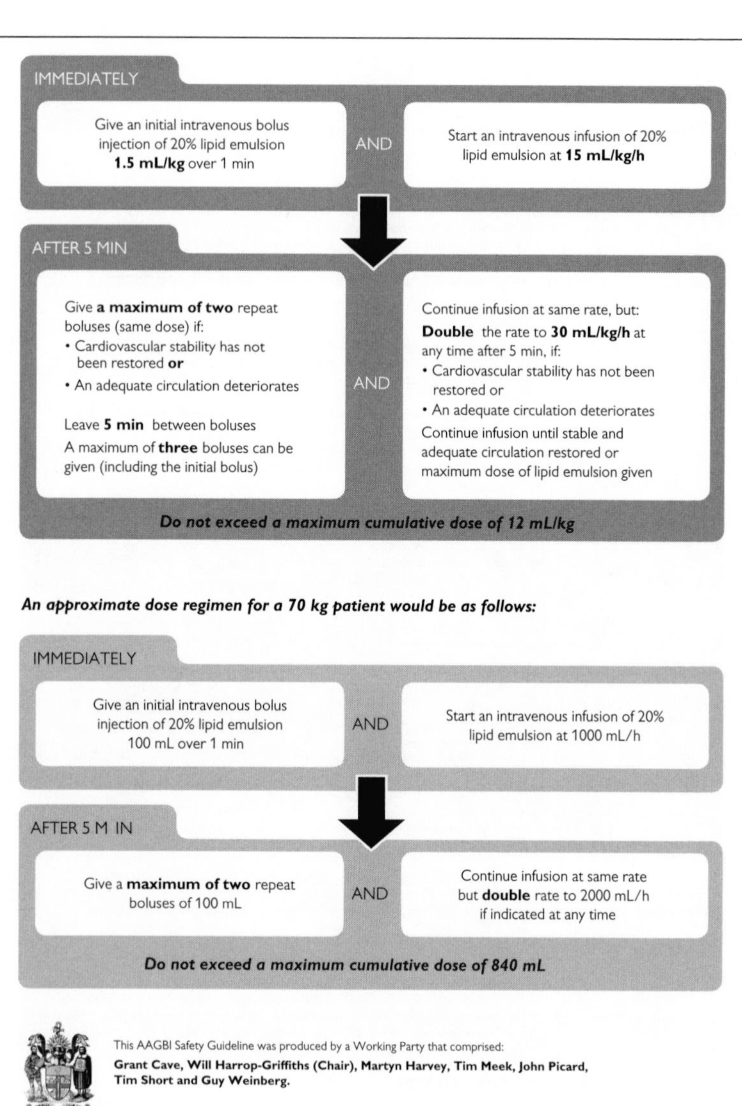

Fig 7.11 Continued

Lipid emulsion is given as a bolus, followed by an infusion. The initial bolus of 1.5 mL/kg is given over 60 s and should be followed by an infusion of 15 mL/kg/h.

If the patient does not improve, the bolus dose can be repeated up to two times at 5 min intervals, and the infusion rate can be doubled to 30 mL/kg/h. The infusion should be continued until the patient is stable or the maximum dose of 12 mL/kg is reached.

7.9 Adult advanced life support

Cardiac arrest is an uncommon event in theatre, but the anaesthetist is commonly called to assist in the management of arrested patients around the hospital, including assisting in stabilizing or transferring them after successful resuscitation.

7.9.1 Adult advanced life support: the Universal Algorithm

ALS is based around the Universal Algorithm, reproduced in Fig 7.12. This approach is standardized across Europe and is taught to providers from a wide variety of professional backgrounds.

7.9.1.1 *Step 1: look for signs of life*

After ensuring that the environment is safe approach the patient and assess their level of responsiveness. If the patient is responsive it implies that they must have a cardiac output and spontaneous respiratory effort.

If the patient is unresponsive look for chest movement to indicate breathing and feel for a carotid pulse. Note that a patient in cardiac arrest may make abnormal gasping movements—'agonal breaths'—but these are not normal chest movements and if any doubt exists continue with life support.

Remember that providing ALS requires a great deal of assistance, so call for help as soon as possible. This may be as simple as shouting for assistance or pressing an emergency buzzer. The team leader must make sure a cardiac arrest call has been made at the earliest opportunity.

7.9.1.2 *Step 2: basic life support*

Once a diagnosis of cardiac arrest has been made, CPR must commence without delay. The responder places both hands, one on top of the other, in the middle of the chest and compresses the chest to a depth of about 5–6 cm. Compressions should be delivered at a rate of 100–120 compressions/min.

After the delivery of 30 compressions, two breaths must be administered. In out-of-hospital arrests, with limited equipment, this may require mouth-to-mouth ventilation, but this is undesirable as it delivers a low inspired oxygen concentration. In hospital, there should be 'pocket-masks' immediately available in all clinical areas. These are both aesthetically more acceptable and also often provide a means of connecting an enriched oxygen supply to the mask. A pocket-mask still requires the provider to give mouth-to-mask breaths.

The best means of providing breaths in a resuscitation situation is using a self-inflating bag. Although the bag can be used without a gas supply, it should be connected to an oxygen flowmeter at the earliest opportunity, as when connected to a high-flow supply it can provide around 80% oxygen.

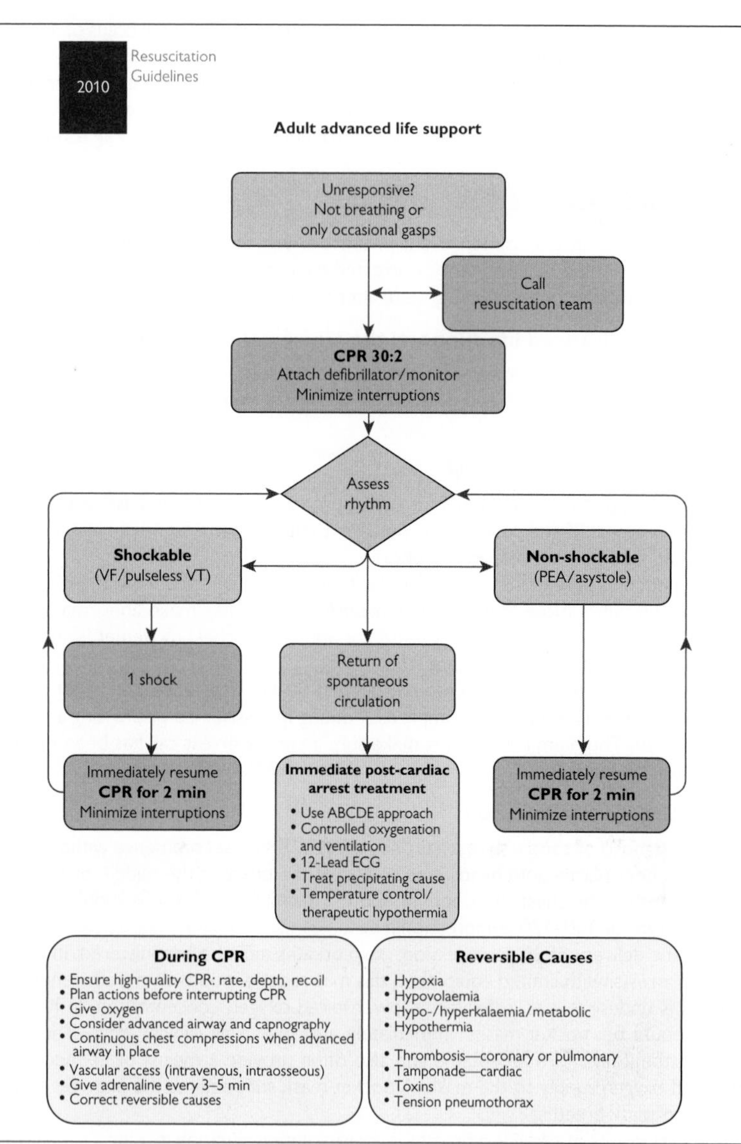

Fig 7.12 The ALS Universal Algorithm (2010).

Regardless of the method of delivering breaths, the rescuer is aiming to provide sufficient volume to cause the chest to rise. Excessively large, fast, or forceful breaths are more likely to inflate the stomach, which increases the risk of regurgitation and can cause respiratory impairment.

CPR continues with this 30:2 ratio until a defibrillator can be connected. It is important to minimize any interruptions in CPR as far as possible; ideally, the only time CPR should not be ongoing is when the rhythm is being checked, or a shock is actually delivered by the defibrillator.

7.9.1.3 *Step 3: connect defibrillator*

As soon as it becomes available, the defibrillator should be connected to the patient. Most clinical areas use hands-free adhesive pads to connect to the patient. One pad is placed to the right of the sternum, while the other is placed in the left axilla. Care should be taken with pad placement if the chest is wet or there are metal implants (including pacemakers) present between the pads. If necessary, pads can be placed on the front and back of the chest. CPR need not pause to place the pads on the patient.

Once the defibrillator pads have been applied, the defibrillator should be switched on. Most modern defibrillators will display the rhythm recorded by the pads on screen by default.

CPR must now be paused to make an assessment of the rhythm. The team leader must decide if the rhythm is shockable or non-shockable. As soon as the rhythm has been diagnosed, CPR should restart.

7.9.1.4 *Step 4a: shockable rhythms*

If the rhythm is ventricular fibrillation (VF) (see Fig 7.13) or pulseless ventricular tachycardia (VT) (see Fig 7.14), a defibrillation shock should be applied without further delay.

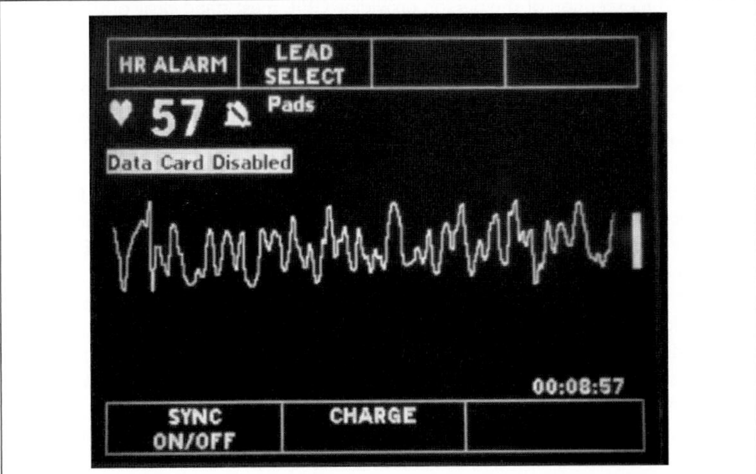

Fig 7.13 A VF rhythm. A short video sequence illustrating VF is available in the video appendix. Please note this video has no audio.

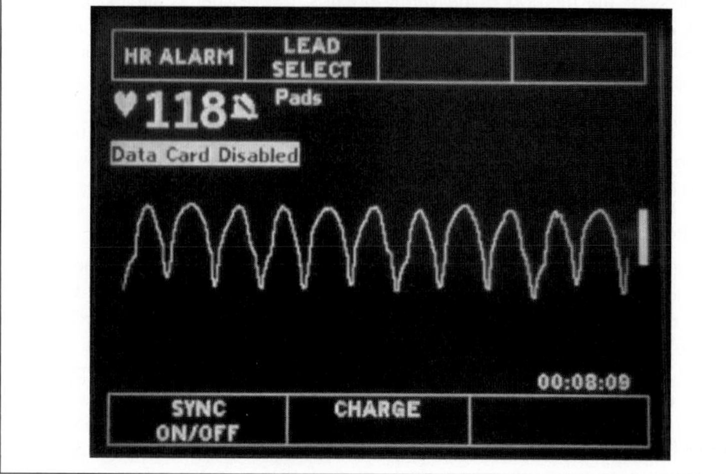

Fig 7.14 A pulseless VT rhythm. A short video sequence illustrating VT is available in the video appendix. Please note this video has no audio.

Current recommendations are for 'hands-on' charging. This means that CPR should continue while the defibrillator is being charged, although all other members of the team must still stand clear and oxygen must still be removed.

To perform this safely there must be good communication and trust between all members of the team. The team leader should brief all the team members and everyone, with the exception of the person providing CPR, must stand clear of the patient.

The provider responsible for the defibrillator should now charge the device and warn all other members of the team (except the CPR provider) to stand clear.

Most defibrillators in current use deliver a 'biphasic' shock. The waveform of these shocks varies from manufacturer to manufacturer, therefore shock energy depends on the defibrillator being used. If there is uncertainty regarding what the appropriate shock energy should be, the highest setting for the machine should be selected.

When the machine has been charged and is ready to deliver a shock the CPR provider must then stand completely clear while the shock is delivered. As soon as the shock has been given CPR restarts without pausing to check for a pulse. CPR should only stop if there are obvious signs of life.

After 2 min of CPR, the team should pause so the rhythm can be reassessed and another decision about defibrillation made.

Adrenaline (1 mg, as 10 mL of a 1:10 000 solution; see Section 2.5.1.3) is given after the third shock and then after each alternate shock thereafter. A dose interval of 3–5 min is desirable.

Amiodarone in a dose of 300 mg is also given after the third shock but is not repeated.

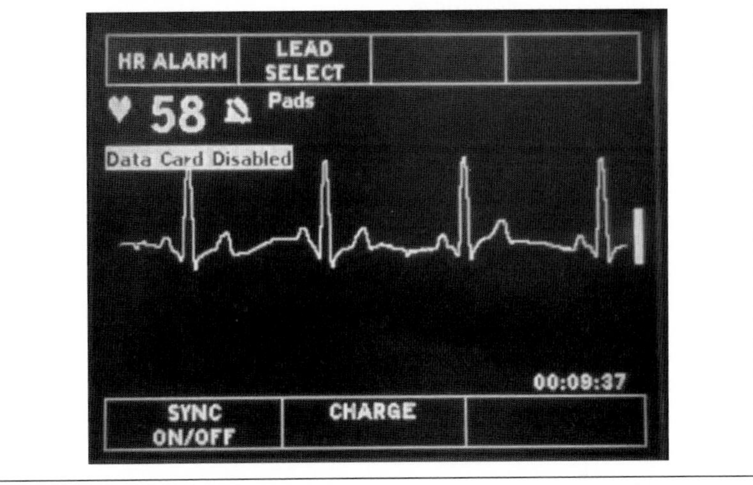

Fig 7.15 An example of a presenting rhythm that, if it occurred during cardiac arrest, would represent a pulseless electrical activity. A short video sequence illustrating such a rhythm is available in the video appendix. Please note this video has no audio.

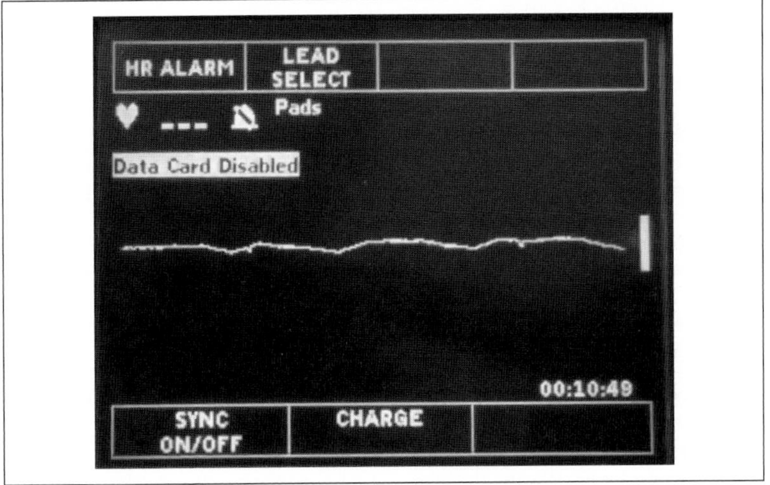

Fig 7.16 An asystole rhythm. A short video sequence illustrating asystole is available in the video appendix. Please note this video has no audio.

7.9.1.5 *Step 4b: non-shockable rhythms*

If the rhythm is neither VF nor VT, then the arrest is non-shockable. The presenting rhythm may be either pulseless electrical activity (see Fig 7.15) or asystole (see Fig 7.16). CPR continues in 2 min cycles until either spontaneous circulation is restored, the rhythm changes to one that is shockable, or the team determines that further resuscitation is no longer appropriate.

In non-shockable arrests, adrenaline (1 mg, as 10 mL of a 1:10000 solution; see Section 2.5.1.3) is given immediately and then in alternate cycles thereafter. A dose interval of 3–5 min is desirable.

7.9.1.6 *Step 5: reversible causes*

During the cardiac arrest, the team leader should give consideration to potentially reversible causes of cardiac arrest. These should be systematically searched for and, if any are found, should be treated immediately.

The potentially reversible causes of cardiac arrest are conveniently remembered as '4Hs' and '4Ts':

- Hypoxia
- Hypovolaemia
- Hypo- or hyperkalaemia
- Hypothermia
- Tension pneumothorax
- Thromboembolism
- Toxic and metabolic causes
- Tamponade (cardiac).

These pathologies should be looked for during any cardiac arrest.

7.9.2 **Post-resuscitation care**

It is vital that, after spontaneous circulation is restored, the team continues to make every effort to stabilize the patient. They are still at high risk of further deterioration, possibly into a repeat cardiac arrest.

If a cardiac rhythm compatible with an output is detected during a rhythm check, or if the patient displays obvious signs of life, the team should pause to check for a carotid pulse.

If a pulse is present the team should conduct an 'A to E' assessment of the patient, checking:

- **Airway:** check the airway is patent, and, if an airway device is present, ensure it is still correctly sited
- **Breathing:** check if the patient is making spontaneous respiratory effort. If not, or if the effort is inadequate, the team will still need to provide some form of respiratory assistance. If the team has sufficient personnel with appropriate skill, draw a blood gas sample

- **Circulation:** assess the pulse rate and rhythm centrally and peripherally. Check capillary refill time and blood pressure
- **Disability:** check the patient's level of consciousness, using the AVPU scale. Remember to check blood glucose (this may be recorded on a blood gas measurement)
- **Exposure:** examine the patient to look for any reversible causes that were not previously apparent. Remember that the patient could have developed new pathology during the arrest, e.g. a pneumothorax.

During the immediate post-arrest phase the anaesthetist will often be required to assist with definitive airway support and with the provision of invasive monitoring via arterial and central venous lines. Most post-arrest patients will need a period of organ support after a cardiac arrest, and a period of therapeutic hypothermia may be appropriate.

Patients may also need to be transferred, either within the hospital (e.g. from the ward to intensive care unit (ICU) or to radiology), or to other institutions for definitive treatment. A senior anaesthetist is well placed to provide support during such movements.

7.9.3 **Human factors in resuscitation**

7.9.3.1 *Situational awareness*

Situational awareness is having knowledge of all of the relevant factors that are contributing to a situation. In a cardiac arrest situation this might include information such as presenting rhythm, duration of arrest, blood results, the patient's past medical history, and the skill mix of the team members.

It is difficult to maintain total situational awareness on an individual basis, particularly when absorbed in technical procedures so it is best, wherever possible, if the person in charge of the team is not also responsible for performing a task like airway management or CPR.

There is a model of 'distributed situational awareness' that relies on all members of the team having knowledge of their particular sphere of responsibility. This depends on good communication of relevant information to the rest of the team. It is good practice to speak up if you think a colleague may not have noticed something important.

7.9.3.2 *The team leader*

One of the most obvious features of a well-run cardiac arrest is the presence of an identifiable team leader. The team leader is the individual who coordinates the actions of the team and ensures that tasks are carried out efficiently. Team members can assist them by only communicating relevant information to prevent 'information overload' and by choosing appropriate times to pass information on.

Most crucially, the team leader should not be responsible for delivering any practical aspect of resuscitation. This is particularly relevant to the anaesthetist; often in resuscitation situations the anaesthetist may be required to manage the airway and therefore would not always make an appropriate choice of leader, at least in the initial stages. Once the airway has been secured and the anaesthetist can focus on the totality of the situation, it may be more appropriate for them to assume the leadership role.

The leader is not necessarily the most senior person present nor need they be medically trained. The most appropriate leader is the person present with most experience of resuscitation; in many situations, this could be a senior nurse or a resuscitation officer.

As they are receiving and assimilating information from each of the team members, the leader should be the person with the most complete understanding of the arrest situation and is therefore the person best placed to make decisions about management, including when to discontinue resuscitation. Team members must, however, be encouraged to discuss any concerns and make alternative suggestions as the situation warrants.

7.9.3.3 *Communication and handover*

Communication in a busy environment should be brief, clear, and timely. Every effort should be made to minimize unnecessary distractions.

When passing messages between team members or communicating with personnel outside of the team, providers should follow the read-back model—the person receiving the information should repeat or summarize the message to confirm it has been correctly heard (see Fig 7.17). This is particularly important when receiving telephone messages, e.g. from hospital laboratories about test results that might inform ongoing management.

When communicating within the team, it is particularly helpful if team members can be addressed by name; this ensures that the attention of the recipient can be gained, and it makes it clear who has responsibility for acting on the message.

Handover of the patient, either in person or via telephone, should follow a structured communication model such as 'SBAR' (see Fig 7.18). SBAR is an acronym for:

- **Situation:** a brief summary of the reason for the call. Identify yourself by name, specialty, and seniority. Confirm the identity of the recipient of the call before presenting a short description of the events precipitating this contact
- **Background:** this is a concise precis of the patient's past history and reason for admission, but only include those details that are relevant to the current situation or that will help inform any decisions
- **Assessment:** this should include any relevant observations that have been made, presented using an ABCDE structure
- **Response:** summarize the actions that have been taken already, and be clear about what is expected or needed from the person that has been called.

A similar model is 'RSVP', which stands for **Reason**, **Story**, **Vitals**, and **Plan**. The information communicated at each stage is equivalent to SBAR. An example of someone using the SBAR system can be seen in Fig 7.19.

7.9.3.4 *Record-keeping*

Accurate records are a crucial component of managing the critically ill patient. Not only does it form a legal account of events, but it will help to inform decisions about ongoing management.

Wherever possible, records should be written contemporaneously. The perception of time during critical events is highly variable. It is difficult to accurately recall when an event occurred or a drug was given afterwards, and it is important to remember that such records may be of crucial importance to outside bodies such as a coroner.

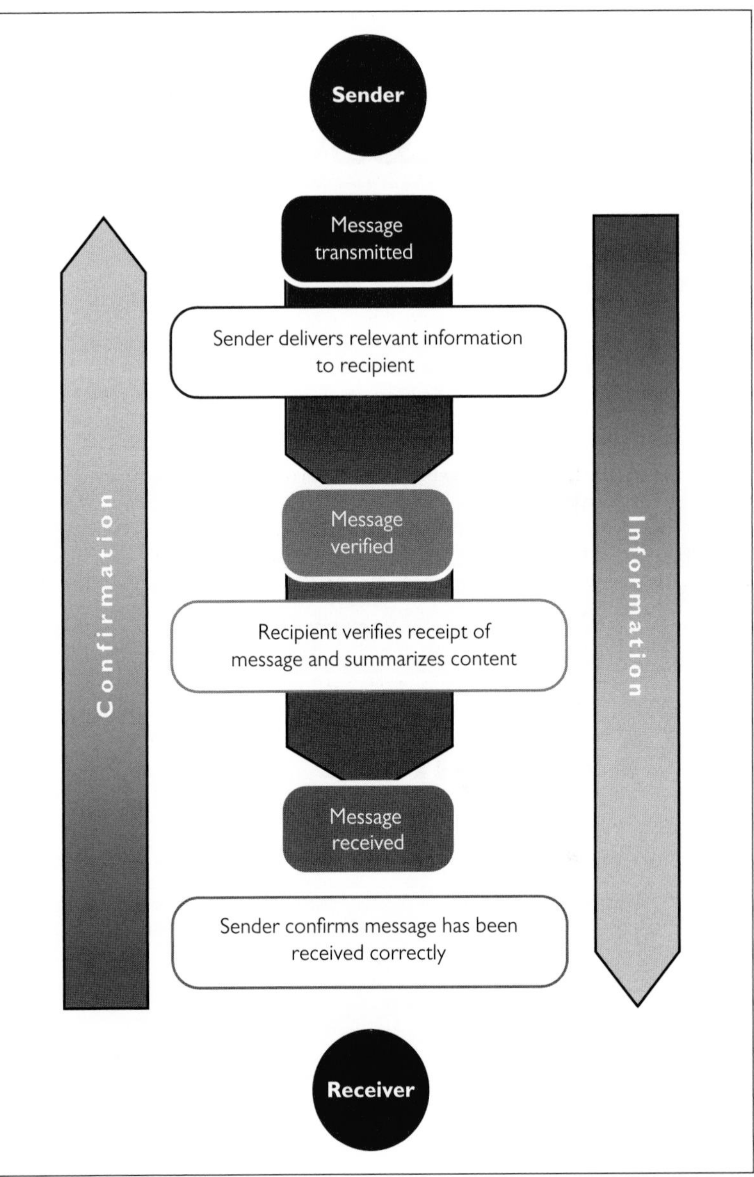

Fig 7.17 An illustration of two-way communication.

Simulation Centre NHS
NHS Trust

S.B.A.R Communication

Communication & assessment framework to use for patients at risk of deterioration

Situation

I am .... (Nurse / Doctor)
Is that .... (Doctor / Specialist) ?
I am calling about .... (Patient's name / location)

- The problem seems to be:
  cardiac / infection /
  neurological / respiratory / renal
- I am not sure what the problem is but the patient is deteriorating

I am concerned that the patient's trigger score is ...

Background

- Reason for admission / recent problems
- Relevant past medical history

The patient's resuscitation status is...

- Not for resuscitation but for full active treatment
- Not for resuscitation
- For resuscitation

Assessment

- Include a full and accurate list of observations and vital signs

My examination findings are:

- A - Airway
- B - Breathing
- C - Circulation
- D - Disability
- E - Exposure

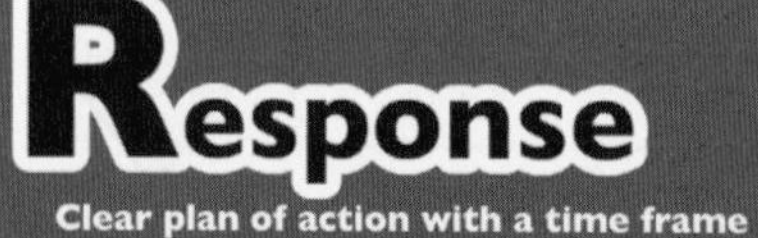

Response

- I have started .... (Treatment)
- Can you recommend any new measures?

Clear plan of action with a time frame

- Please see the patient now, or within .... mins

Any tests needed?

- CXR / ABG / ECG / BC / Others?

Fig 7.18 A poster illustrating the SBAR model of handover communication.

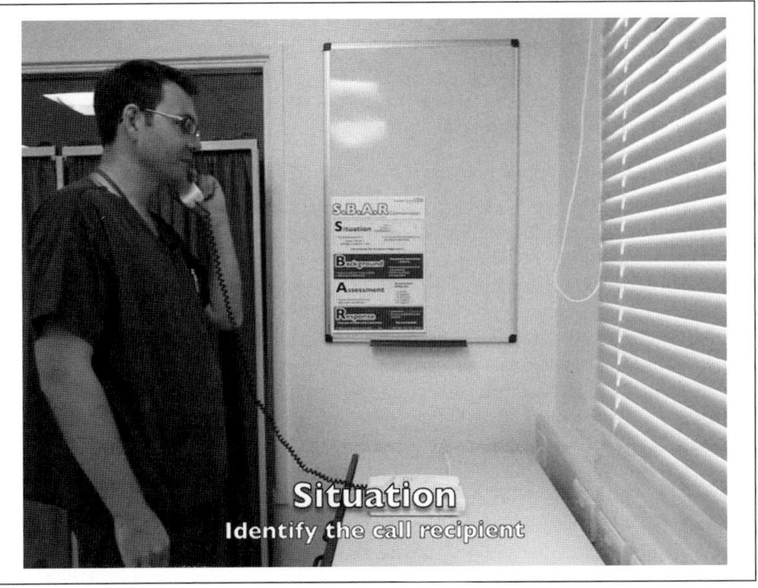

Fig 7.19 Handover of the patient, either in person or via telephone, should follow a structured communication model such as 'SBAR' where the anaesthetist outlines the Situation, Background, Assessment, and Response. A short video sequence illustrating an SBAR handover is available in the video appendix.

Although early in an arrest there may not be enough personnel available to assign someone to record-keeping, it is extremely helpful if a person can devote their attention to 'real-time' record-keeping. This individual is also well placed to time cardiac arrest cycles and drug dose intervals.

7.10 Tachycardia and bradycardia

Arrhythmias are common in anaesthetic practice although, fortunately, few require treatment. The approach to the patient with a pathological arrhythmia is the same, whether the patient is under anaesthesia or not; patients should be assessed in an 'A to E' manner, and all patients should receive supplemental oxygen. IV access should be established and monitoring commenced.

The patient should be examined for the following adverse signs:

- Clinical evidence of shock
- Syncope
- Signs of myocardial ischaemia
- Signs of heart failure.

7.10.1 **Tachycardia**

Guidelines for the management of tachycardia produced by the Resuscitation Council (UK) are reproduced in Fig 7.20.

The tachycardic patient who demonstrates adverse signs would be considered unstable and would require DC cardioversion.

7.10.1.1 *Treating the unstable patient*

A DC shock is delivered in a similar manner to defibrillation, with some crucial differences. Importantly, the shock must be synchronized to the R wave, because a shock delivered on a T wave could induce VF. Synchronization is achieved by pressing the 'sync' button on the defibrillator. The defibrillator then marks each QRS complex, and the 'sync' indicator illuminates, as demonstrated in Fig 7.21 and Fig 7.22.

Another important difference is that the tachycardic patient may well be conscious. As delivery of the shock is painful, it is common for patients to require sedation or general anaesthesia to facilitate the treatment. Selecting an appropriate anaesthetic agent and dose can be complicated; generally, shocked patients are more sensitive to anaesthetic agents, so comparatively small doses are often adequate, but the drugs tend to have much slower onset. Always take advice from a senior colleague.

After the patient has been appropriately sedated, the synchronized shock can be delivered. As with defibrillation, all oxygen should be disconnected and team members asked to stand clear. After delivery of the shock, reassess the patient. If they remain unstable, a second and third shock may be indicated.

If, after three shocks, the patient remains unstable, they should receive 300 mg amiodarone over 10–20 min, after which a final shock may be attempted, if required.

7.10.1.2 *Treating the stable patient*

For those tachycardic patients who lack adverse features, medical management forms the first line of treatment.

To decide which drugs are required, decide first if the rhythm is broad or narrow complex and then if it is regular or irregular.

- **Broad complex, regular rhythm:** likely VT, requiring amiodarone treatment; less commonly, a supraventricular tachycardia (SVT) with abnormal conduction. If the patient is known to have a pre-existing bundle-branch block, treat as a narrow complex, regular rhythm
- **Broad complex, irregular rhythm:** likely torsade-de-pointe or an unusual presentation of AF. These rhythms are more complex and will require expert intervention. Treatment may include magnesium (for torsade) or amiodarone (for AF)
- **Narrow complex, regular rhythm:** likely SVT, requiring initial management with vagal manoeuvres such as carotid sinus massage or a Valsalva manoeuvre. Adenosine is indicated if the rhythm is not controlled. Adenosine must be given as fast boluses, starting with 6 mg, then increasing to 12 mg for the second and third doses (if required). Adenosine causes transient atrioventricular (AV) node block, and the patient will experience significant, but short-lived, discomfort. If sinus rhythm is not restored, expert help should be sought

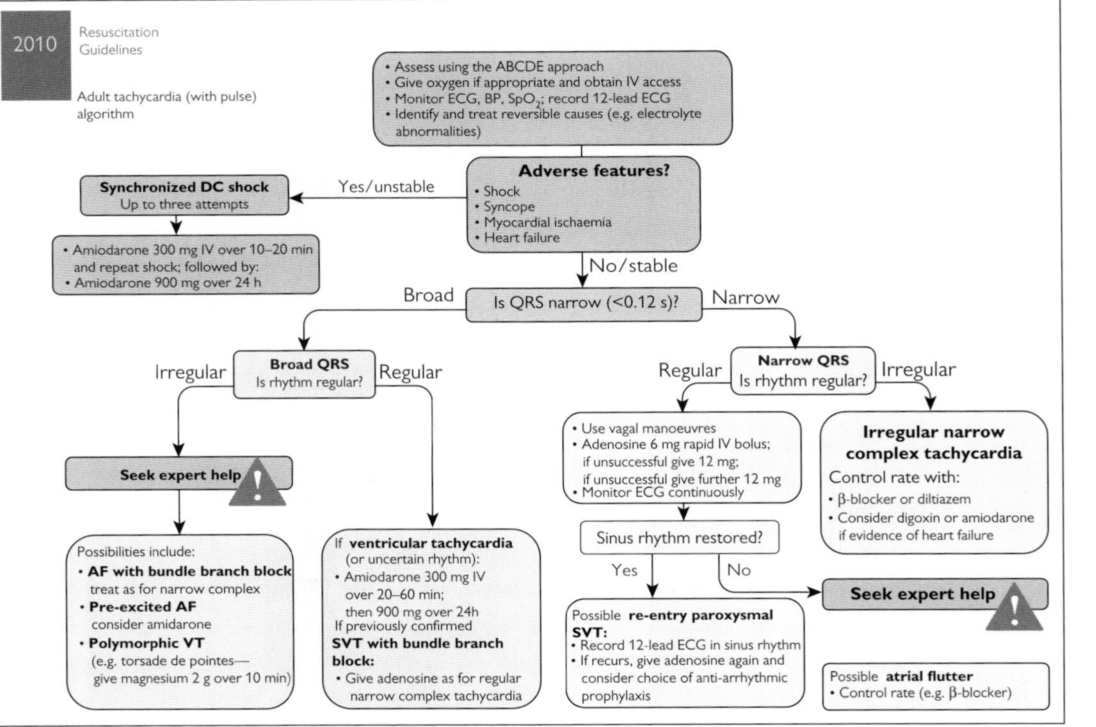

2010
Resuscitation Guidelines
Adult tachycardia (with pulse) algorithm
• Assess using the ABCDE approach
• Give oxygen if appropriate and obtain IV access
• Monitor ECG, BP, SpO_2; record 12-lead ECG
• Identify and treat reversible causes (e.g. electrolyte abnormalities)
Adverse features?
• Shock
• Syncope
• Myocardial ischaemia
• Heart failure
Yes/unstable
Synchronized DC shock
Up to three attempts
• Amiodarone 300 mg IV over 10–20 min and repeat shock; followed by:
• Amiodarone 900 mg over 24 h
No/stable
Is QRS narrow (<0.12 s)?
Broad
Narrow
Broad QRS
Is rhythm regular?
Irregular
Regular
Seek expert help
Possibilities include:
• AF with bundle branch block treat as for narrow complex
• Pre-excited AF consider amidarone
• Polymorphic VT (e.g. torsade de pointes— give magnesium 2 g over 10 min)
If ventricular tachycardia (or uncertain rhythm):
• Amiodarone 300 mg IV over 20–60 min; then 900 mg over 24h
If previously confirmed SVT with bundle branch block:
• Give adenosine as for regular narrow complex tachycardia
Narrow QRS
Is rhythm regular?
Regular
Irregular
• Use vagal manoeuvres
• Adenosine 6 mg rapid IV bolus; if unsuccessful give 12 mg; if unsuccessful give further 12 mg
• Monitor ECG continuously
Sinus rhythm restored?
Yes
No
Possible re-entry paroxysmal SVT:
• Record 12-lead ECG in sinus rhythm
• If recurs, give adenosine again and consider choice of anti-arrhythmic prophylaxis
Irregular narrow complex tachycardia
Control rate with:
• β-blocker or diltiazem
• Consider digoxin or amiodarone if evidence of heart failure
Seek expert help
Possible atrial flutter
• Control rate (e.g. β-blocker)

Fig 7.20 Algorithm for the management of tachycardia (2010).
Reproduced with the kind permission of the Resuscitation Council (UK).

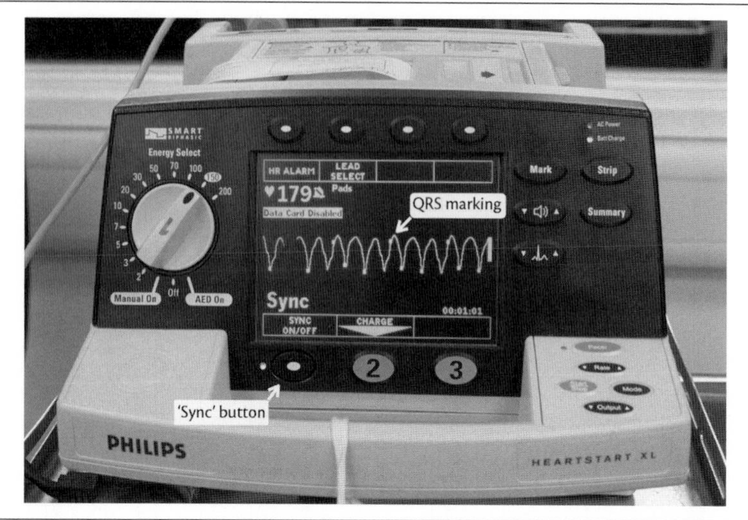

Fig 7.21 The 'sync' button on this Philips HeartStart defibrillator can be seen below and to the left of the screen. The screen displays 'SYNC ON/OFF' just above the control.

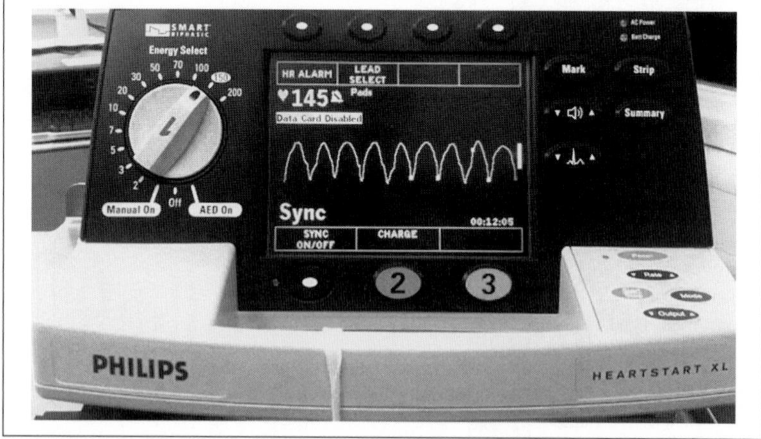

Fig 7.22 Synchronization of a shock to the R wave is achieved by pressing the 'sync' button on the defibrillator. The defibrillator then marks each QRS complex, and the 'sync' indicator illuminates. A short video demonstrating how the defibrillator marks QRS complexes after the 'sync' button has been pressed is available in the video appendix. Note that a green LED flashes next to the button, and the screen displays 'Sync' to confirm the defibrillator mode. Please note this video has no audio.

- **Narrow complex, irregular rhythm:** likely AF, requiring either rate control or rhythm control. Rate control is indicated if the AF is not known to be of new onset and can be achieved with β-blockade, calcium channel blockers, or digoxin. It is possible to chemically cardiovert the patient using amiodarone, which is useful if the AF is of new onset but may cause embolization of an atrial thrombus if the AF is long-standing.

7.10.2 Bradycardia

Guidelines for the management of bradycardia produced by the Resuscitation Council (UK) are reproduced in Fig 7.23.

The unstable bradycardic patient requires treatment, initially with atropine (see Section 2.5.2.1). A dose of 500 micrograms is given and the response evaluated.

If a satisfactory response is achieved and the patient is not at risk of further deterioration, they can be observed in a suitable clinical environment.

If the response is not satisfactory the patient will require further doses of atropine, repeated every 5 min, up to a maximum of 3 mg, if required.

Transcutaneous pacing may be a useful interim measure while arrangements are made for transvenous pacing. Sedation will be required for transcutaneous pacing in the conscious patient, as it is uncomfortable. Unlike defibrillation, oxygen can be administered while the pacer is running and it is safe to touch the patient.

7.11 Malignant hyperthermia

Malignant hyperthermia, also known as malignant hyperpyrexia or MH, is an autosomal dominant inherited abnormality that predisposes carriers to a hypermetabolic state triggered by exposure to certain agents. The condition is rare and affects around 1 in 200 000 people in the UK. Guidelines for its management have been produced by the AAGBI (see Fig 7.24).

MH trigger agents include all volatile anaesthetic agents (see Section 2.3) and suxamethonium (see Section 2.4.2.1). IV induction agents, like propofol or thiopental (see Section 2.2), are safe, as are all non-depolarizing neuromuscular-blocking agents (see Section 2.4.1).

7.11.1 Presentation

The hyperthermia for which the condition is named is a late sign. The diagnosis is suggested by masseter spasm after administration of suxamethonium. Early signs also include an unexplained tachycardia or progressive rise in end-tidal CO_2. MH patients often develop cardiovascular instability and muscle rigidity.

7.11.2 Initial treatment

Initial treatment is supportive. Trigger agents should be stopped and, if a volatile agent has been used, the vaporizer should be removed and a new breathing circuit attached. Give the patient 100% oxygen at high flows to flush out any remaining volatile in the system.

Summon help immediately and inform the surgeon; stop surgery, if possible. Maintain anaesthesia by propofol boluses or an infusion.

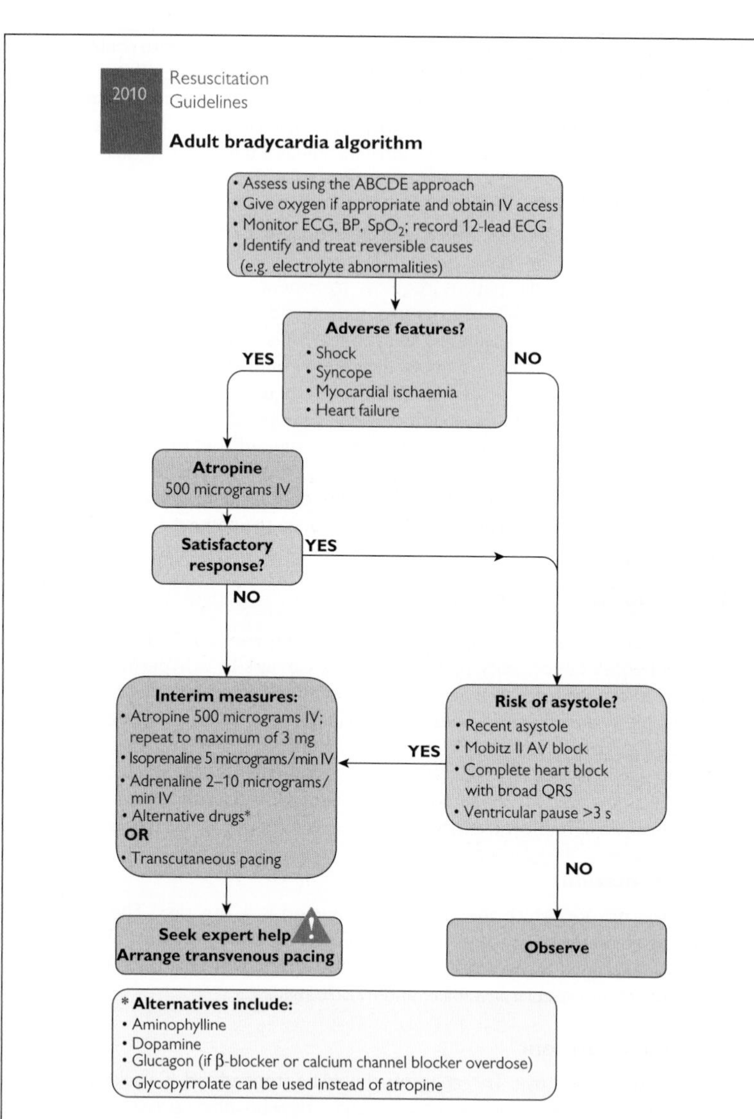

Fig 7.23 Algorithm for the management of bradycardia (2010).

Malignant Hyperthermia Crisis

AAGBI Safety Guideline

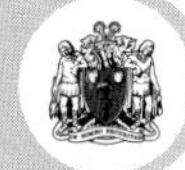

Onest can be within minutes of induction or may be insidious. The standard operating procedure below is intended to ease the burden of managing this rare, but life-threatening, emergency.

1 Recognition

- Unexplained increase in $EtCO_2$ **AND**
- Unexplained tachycardia **AND**
- Unexplained increase in oxygen requirement
  (previous uneventful anaesthesia does **not** rule out MH)
- Temperature changes are a late sign

2 Immediate management

- **STOP** all trigger agents
- **CALL FOR HELP.** Allocate specific tasks (action plan in MH kit)
- Install clean breathing system and **HYPERVENTILATE** with **100% O_2 high flow**
- Maintain anaesthesia with intravenous agent
- **ABANDON/FINISH** surgery as soon as possible
- Muscle relaxation with non-depolarizing neuromuscular-blocking drug

3 Monitoring and treatment

- Give **dantrolene**
- Initiate active **cooling** avoiding vasoconstriction
- **TREAT:**
  - **Hyperkalaemia:** calcium chloride, glucose/insulin, $NaHCO_3^-$
  - **Arrhythmias:** magnesium/amiodarone/metoprolol
    AVOID calcium channel blockers—interaction with dantrolene
  - **Metabolic acidosis:** hyperventilate, $NaHCO_3^-$
  - **Myoglobinaemia:** forced alkaline diuresis (mannitol/furosemide + $NaHCO_3^-$); may require renal replacement therapy later
  - **DIC:** FFP, cryoprecipitiate, platelets
- Check plasma CK as soon as able

DANTROLENE
2.5 mg/kg immediate IV bolus.
Repeat 1 mg/kg boluses as required to max 10 mg/kg

For a 70 kg adult

- **Initial bolus: nine vials dantrolene** 20 mg (each vial mixed with 60 mL sterile water)
- Further boluses of four vials dantrolene 20 mg repeated up to 7 times.

Continuous monitoring
Core and peripheral temperature
$EtCO_2$
SpO_2
ECG
Invasive blood pressure
CVP

Repeated bloods
ABG
U&Es (potassium)
FBC (haematocrit/platelets)
Coagulation

4 Follow-up

- Continue monitoring on ICU, repeat dantrolene as necessary
- Monitor for acute kidney injury and compartment syndrome
- Repeat CK
- Consider alternative diagnoses (sepsis, phaeochromocytoma, thyroid storm, myopathy)
- Counsel patient and family members
- Refer to MH unit (see contact details below)

The UK MH Investigation Unit, Academic Unit of Anaesthesia, Clinical Sciences Building, Leeds Teaching Hospitals NHS Trust, Leeds LS9 7TF. Direct line: 0113 206 5270. Fax: 0113 206 4140. Emergency Hotline: 07947 609601 (usually available outside office hours). Alternatively, contact Prof P Hopkins, Dr E Watkins or Dr P Gupta through hospital switchboard: 0113 243 3144.

Fig 7.24 Guidelines for the management of MH (2011).

Cool the patient—stop any forced-air warming; remove blankets, and apply ice packs around the axillae and groins. Infuse cold fluids IV, and cold bladder or peritoneal lavage may be beneficial.

Check a blood gas sample for acidosis and hyperkalaemia; an otherwise unexplained metabolic acidosis confirms the diagnosis. Correct metabolic abnormalities where necessary. Invasive blood pressure and central venous pressure monitoring may be required.

Blood samples should be sent for creatine kinase analysis and clotting, and a urine sample sent for myoglobin. Rhabdomyolysis may cause acute renal failure, which may require renal replacement therapy. IV fluids, with or without diuretics to promote diuresis, are required in the event of myoglobinaemia.

7.11.3 **Definitive treatment**

The definitive treatment of MH is with dantrolene. Dantrolene reduces calcium release from the muscle cell sarcoplasmic reticulum, decreasing muscle contraction and therefore correcting the underlying metabolic abnormality. It should be given as soon as possible after the diagnosis has been made.

Dantrolene is supplied in vials containing 20 mg of dantrolene powder, and each vial should be made up to 60 mL. It is not particularly water-soluble and takes a lot of time to mix up, so it should be requested early and a person may need to be dedicated to preparing the drug.

Dantrolene is given as an initial bolus of 2.5 mg/kg, with doses of 1 mg/kg repeated up to a maximum total dose of 10 mg/kg. After an event patients should be monitored in the intensive care unit (ICU). Dantrolene can produce skeletal muscle weakness and respiratory embarrassment, and MH symptoms can recur. Acute kidney injury can occur, and renal replacement therapy may be needed.

All patients with a suspected episode of MH should be referred to the National MH Investigation Unit in Leeds for testing and follow-up.

7.12 **Self-assessment questions**

Answer either true or false for each of the following questions. The answers can be found in Appendix 2.

1. **Which of the following should be performed after a failed intubation during RSI?**
   - A. Call for help
   - B. Make no more than three attempts to intubate the patient
   - C. Give a further dose of muscle relaxant to make sure the suxamethonium does not wear off
   - D. Oxygenate the patient by mask ventilation
   - E. Take steps to minimize delays, and ensure surgery starts as soon as possible

2. **The capnograph waveform appears as in Fig 7.25. What are possible causes?**
   - A. Disconnection of the breathing circuit
   - B. Major haemorrhage
   - C. Anaphylaxis

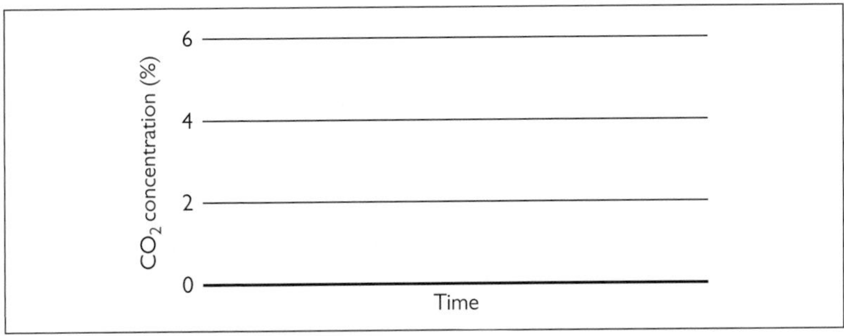

Fig 7.25 Capnograph waveform.

D. Obstruction of a tracheal tube
E. Pneumothorax

3. Which of the following might cause raised airway pressures?

A. Disconnection of the breathing circuit
B. Major haemorrhage
C. Anaphylaxis
D. Obstruction of a tracheal tube
E. Pneumothorax

4. Which drugs should be given to a patient suffering from anaphylaxis?

A. IM adrenaline
B. Hydrocortisone
C. Fluid challenge with IV colloid solution
D. Chloramphenicol
E. Ipratropium bromide

5. Please look at the cardiac rhythm in Fig 7.26:

A. This rhythm is AF
B. This rhythm would be best treated by DC cardioversion
C. This rhythm may be associated with cardiac arrest
D. If this rhythm appeared on a cardiac monitor, the patient will always be pulseless
E. IV adrenaline would be the treatment of first choice if the patient were pulseless

6. Please look at the cardiac rhythm in Fig 7.26. What treatment(s) would be required if you confirm the patient is pulseless?

A. Immediate defibrillation
B. Adrenaline if two shocks had already been given
C. Amiodarone if three shocks had already been given

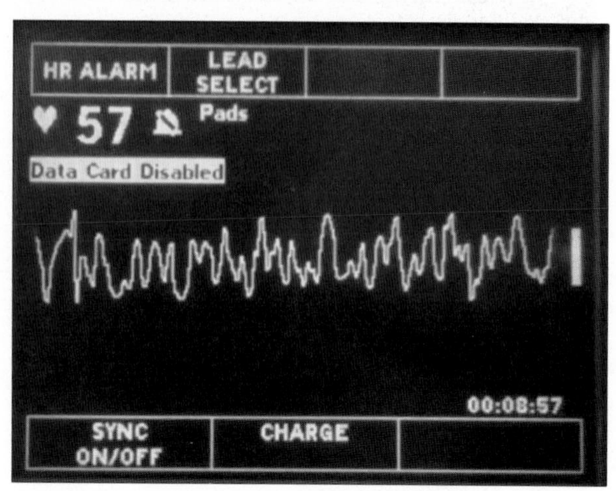

Fig 7.26 Cardiac rhythm.

D. Atropine if three shocks had already been given
E. Transcutaneous pacing may be required

7. Which of these solutions contain exactly 1 mg of adrenaline?
    A. 1 mL of a 1:10 000 solution
    B. 0.5 mL of a 1:1000 solution
    C. 1 mL of a 1:1000 solution
    D. 5 mL of a 1:10 000 solution
    E. 10 mL of a 1:10 000 solution

8. Please look at the rhythm in Fig 7.27. It was recorded in a patient with a heart rate of 120 and a blood pressure of 70. The patient has chest pain and is breathless.
    A. Defibrillation is required
    B. The patient requires sedation or anaesthesia to permit DC cardioversion
    C. Drug therapy, using amiodarone, would be the first line of management

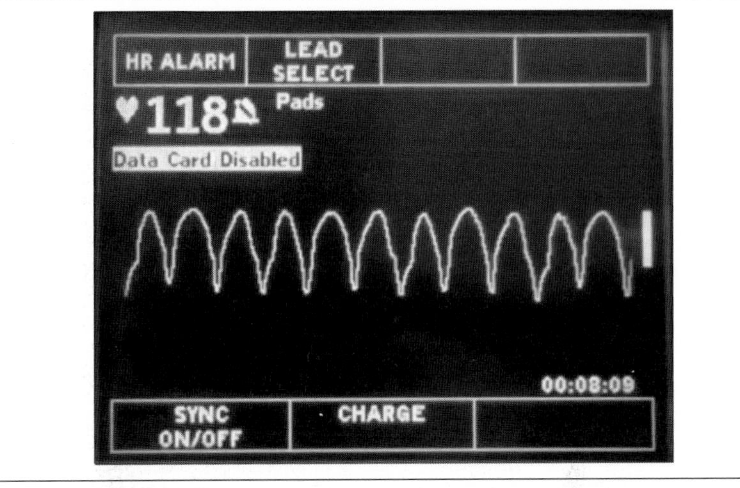

Fig 7.27 Cardiac rhythm.

D. Digoxin could be used to gain rate control

E. Amiodarone has no role in the management of this rhythm

9. **Carotid sinus massage would be indicated in the treatment of which of the following rhythm disturbances?**

   A. A stable patient with a sinus tachycardia

   B. An unstable patient with a narrow complex tachycardia

   C. A stable patient with fast AF

   D. An unstable patient with a sinus tachycardia

   E. A stable patient with an atrial tachycardia

10. **Which of the following statements about MH are true?**

   A. Propofol is never a trigger of MH

   B. Hyperthermia is an early feature of MH

   C. Definitive treatment is with intralipid

   D. Tryptase samples are used in the follow-up of MH

   E. The National MH Investigation Unit is based in Leeds

Appendix 1

Glossary

Absolute pressure

Absolute pressure describes pressure measurements quoted relative to a perfect vacuum. This means that a completely empty gas cylinder would have an absolute pressure of approximately 100 kPa, reflecting atmospheric pressure.

Index: see Section 1.2.3: Pressure gauges

Related glossary terms: Gauge pressure; Pascal

Adrenaline

Adrenaline is a potent inotrope and chronotrope used in the emergency management of anaphylaxis, cardiac arrest, and in the pharmacological management of symptomatic bradycardia. It also has a role by continuous infusion for circulatory support of patients with intractable shock. Nebulized, it has a role in upper airway obstruction.

The dose and route vary by indication; for anaphylaxis, an IM dose of 500 micrograms is generally used outside of theatre. Very small IV doses (up to 50 micrograms) may be indicated in the treatment of in-theatre anaphylaxis, but the scope for dose errors is significant.

In cardiac arrest, doses of 1 mg IV are given as a bolus.

Index: see Section 2.5.1.3: Adrenaline; see Section 7.7: Anaphylaxis; see Section 7.9: Adult advanced life support

Related glossary terms: Chronotrope; Inotrope

American Society of Anesthesiologists

The ASA is an American society that exists to further the academic and clinical practice of anaesthesia in the United States. The ASA Committee on Professional Education Oversight has responsibilities for graduate education and accreditation roughly analogous to the UK Royal College of Anaesthetists. The Division of Scientific Affairs is responsible for continuing medical education and is comparable to the AAGBI in the UK.

Index: see Section 3.2.4: ASA grading

Related glossary terms: Association of Anaesthetists of Great Britain and Ireland

Ametop®

A topical LA gel consisting of amethocaine; it is used mainly in paediatric anaesthesia to reduce cannula insertion pain. As with EMLA®, it is applied with a dressing. Onset is over approximately 30 min.

Index: see Section 2.8: Local anaesthetics

Related glossary terms: EMLA®

Anaesthetic agent potency

Potency is an indicator of the potential for a drug to exert a clinical effect. In the context of anaesthetic agents, potency is reflected in MAC value—a drug with lower MAC is more potent than one with higher, as it takes less of the agent to exert the clinical effect. Potency of inhalational agents is related to lipid solubility. Isoflurane (MAC 1.1) is more potent than sevoflurane (MAC 2.0), and both are more potent than desflurane (MAC 6.35).

Note that speed of onset is related to water solubility but not related to potency.

Index: see Section 2.3: Inhalational anaesthetic agents

Related glossary terms: Anaesthetic agent solubility; Desflurane; Isoflurane; Sevoflurane

Anaesthetic agent solubility

The solubility of an inhalational anaesthetic agent in blood is described by its blood:gas (B:G) partition coefficient, reflecting the mass of an agent that can dissolve in blood.

The clinical effect of an inhalational agent is exerted by the partial pressure of the agent in the blood (which drives diffusion into the brain), so an insoluble agent will reach a higher partial pressure more quickly than a soluble one. This means that, paradoxically, an insoluble agent has a faster onset/offset time than a soluble agent does.

Higher partition coefficients reflect more soluble agents, so isoflurane (B:G 1.4) is more soluble than sevoflurane (B:G 0.7), and both are more soluble than desflurane (B:G 0.45).

Note that solubility in blood is not related to potency.

Index: see Section 2.3: Inhalational anaesthetic agents

Related glossary terms: Anaesthetic agent potency; Desflurane; Isoflurane; Sevoflurane

APL valve

The APL valve is a feature of most anaesthetic breathing circuits. It can be set between 0 cmH_2O and 70 cmH_2O to control the pressure within the breathing circuit. It is generally set between 0 and 5 cmH_2O for spontaneous ventilation and between 15 and 30 cmH_2O in manual ventilation. Although it is rarely necessary to exceed these pressures, it is sometime required when using certain older types of ventilators (like a Penlon Nuffield 200) that use their own pressure-limiting systems or when manually ventilating a patient with a large face mask leak.

If the valve is accidentally closed when connected to the patient, the reservoir bag will distend, limiting pressures to around 40 cmH_2O until the bag fills, as a protective measure to delay the application of the highest pressure to the airway.

Index: see Section 1.2.9: Breathing circuits; see Section 7.5.3: Laryngospasm

Arm:brain circulation time

This represents the time taken for a drug to transit from a peripheral injection site to the brain. The duration can vary depending on cardiac output, and is prolonged in low output states.

Index: see Section 2.2: Intravenous anaesthetic agents

Association of Anaesthetists of Great Britain and Ireland

The AABGI is a professional body representing over 10 000 anaesthetists across the UK and Republic of Ireland. The AAGBI was founded by Sir Ivan Magill and Dr Henry Featherstone in 1932. The AAGBI exists to encourage ongoing improvement in academic and clinical anaesthesia. The Association produces and updates a number of clinical guidelines to do with all aspects of anaesthetic practice and arranges a number of academic seminars at its premises in Central London and around the country.

Index: see Section 1.4: Monitoring equipment; see Section 1.5: Machine checks

Atracurium

Atracurium is a non-depolarizing benzylisoquinolinium neuromuscular blocker, given in a dose of 0.5 mg/kg. It produces muscle relaxation in 3 min. Atracurium can trigger histamine release, which may be associated with bronchoconstriction, hypotension, and skin reactions.

Muscle relaxation lasts for 30 min and is reversible with neostigmine and glycopyrrolate.

In part, metabolism is by spontaneous Hofmann elimination, so the duration of action is not significantly prolonged in renal or hepatic failure.

Index: see Section 2.4.1.1: Atracurium; see Chapter 3: Planning for general anaesthesia; see Chapter 4: Routine induction of general anaesthesia; see Chapter 5: The rapid sequence induction

Related glossary terms: Hofmann elimination; neostigmine and glycopyrrolate; non-depolarizing muscle relaxant

Atropine

Atropine is a competitive antagonist at muscarinic acetylcholine receptors. It is used most commonly to treat bradycardia, typically in doses of 300–600 mg (up to a maximum of 3 mg). It can cross the blood–brain barrier, causing confusion. Other anticholinergic side effects include dry eyes, dry mouth, blurred vision, decreased gastric motility, and urinary retention.
Index: see Section 2.5.2.1: Atropine; see Section 7.10.2: Bradycardia

Bobbin

The bobbin is the small spindle that floats within the gas stream of a flowmeter. Bobbins are designed to spin as they float, so it should be obvious if the bobbin has become stuck. They are generally made from metal so that static electricity (which can cause the bobbin to stick) can be conducted away through earthing strips within the flowmeter tube. Different types of bobbins are read differently. Ball-type bobbins are read from the centre of the ball, whereas the cylindrical bobbins found on most anaesthetic machines are read from the top.
Index: see Section 1.2.5: The flowmeter; see Section 1.5: Machine checks
Related glossary terms: Flowmeter

Bodok seal

A Bodok seal is a neoprene disc, approximately 1 cm in diameter, which helps to provide a gas-tight seal between a cylinder yoke and the anaesthetic machine. The Bodok seal was introduced in the 1950s, along with the pin-index system. Leaks can occur if the seal is damaged or misaligned.
Index: see Section 1.2.2: Gas cylinders
Related glossary terms: Pin-index system

Bougie

A bougie is a long plastic or gum-elastic introducer designed to aid intubation. It is more rigid than most tracheal tubes, and a bend at the tip aids placement between the vocal cords. After siting the bougie in the trachea, a tracheal tube can be railroaded over the top.

Bougies can also be used to exchange airway devices.
Index: see Section 1.5: Machine checks; see Section 7.2: Airway problems at induction

Bourdon gauge

A Bourdon gauge is used to measure high-pressure systems. The gauge is formed from a coiled tube connected to a dial. Gas under pressure fills the tube, which tends to cause the tube to unroll. The degree to which the tube uncoils depends on the pressure of the gas. This movement is displayed by a needle rotating across a dial, upon which is marked a scale from which the pressure can be read (see Fig 8.1).

Frenchman Eugene Bourdon patented the device in 1849.
Index: see Section 1.2.3: Pressure gauges
Related glossary terms: Absolute pressure; Gauge pressure

Boyle's Law

Boyle's Law, first described by physicist Robert Boyle in 1662, describes how the pressure of an ideal gas varies with volume, given constant temperature. It states that, provided temperature does not change, the absolute pressure of a fixed mass of gas is inversely proportional to its volume.
Index: see Section 1.2.2: Gas cylinders
Related glossary terms: Absolute pressure

Breathing circuit

A breathing circuit is a series of components designed to carry gases from the anaesthetic machine to the patient. Breathing circuits can contain various combinations of hoses, valves, a reservoir bag, and a means of connecting to the airway or face mask.

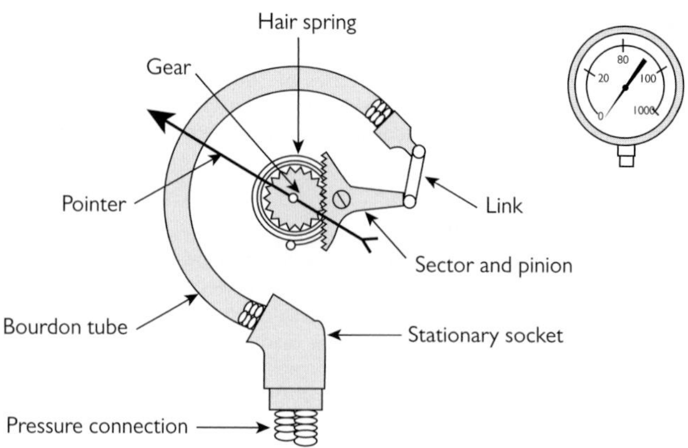

Fig 8.1 An illustration of a Bourdon gauge.
Reproduced by kind permission of Anaesthesia UK.

The performance of breathing circuits varies, depending on the position that fresh gas is introduced to the circuit, relative to the patient and the exhaust valve.
Index: see Section 1.2.7: The common gas outlet; see Section 1.2.9: Breathing circuits; see Section 1.4.5: Anaesthetic agent monitoring; see Chapter 3: Planning for general anaesthesia; see Chapter 4: Routine induction of general anaesthesia; see Chapter 5: The rapid sequence induction; see Section 7.2: Airway problems at induction; see Section 7.3: Loss of capnography waveform; see Section 7.4: High airway pressures
Related glossary terms: Circle breathing system; Breathing circuit; Mapleson C; Mapleson classification; Mapleson D; Mapleson F; Rebreathing

Bupivacaine

Bupivacaine is a long-acting LA agent. The drug is highly protein-bound, meaning that it persists in tissues for longer than other agents. This is useful in that it prolongs clinical effects but also increases the hazards associated with toxic doses.

Bupivacaine is commonly used in peripheral nerve blocks, spinal anaesthetics, and epidural infusions. The preparation used in spinal anaesthesia often contains glucose ('heavy bupivacaine'), which increases the density of the solution, compared to CSF; this aids the drug spread predictably with changes in patient position.

The maximum dose of bupivacaine, for both plain and adrenaline-containing solutions, is 2 mg/kg.
Index: see Section 2.8.2: Bupivacaine; see Section 7.8: Local anaesthetic toxicity
Related glossary terms: Epidural anaesthesia; Local anaesthetics; Spinal anaesthesia

Carotid sinus massage

Carotid sinus massage describes the application of external pressure to the carotid sinus, located at the origin of the internal carotid artery in the neck. Activation of baroreceptors in the sinus results in a reflex bradycardia, which can be useful in terminating narrow complex tachycardias.

It should not be performed on patients with carotid bruit (which should be examined for), and it should only ever be performed unilaterally.
Index: see Section 7.10.1: Tachycardia

Central neuraxial blockade

Two regional anaesthetic techniques are described by the term central neuraxial blockade: spinal and epidural anaesthesia. Central neuraxial blocks can be placed as anaesthetic techniques in their own right or as adjuncts to general anaesthesia.

Epidural analgesia is the provision of pain relief using LAs and/or opioids administered via epidural catheter, without producing complete anaesthesia.

Index: see Section 2.8: Local anaesthetics; see Chapter 6: Central neuraxial blockade

Chemoreceptor trigger zone

The CTZ is situated in the area postrema of the medulla, along the walls of the fourth ventricle. It is outside of the blood–brain barrier and therefore responds to blood-borne agents.

It is richly supplied with dopaminergic (D_2) and serotonergic ($5\text{-}HT_3$) receptors.

Index: see Section 2.7: Antiemetics

Related glossary terms: Metoclopramide; Ondansetron; Vomiting centre

Chronotrope

A chronotrope is a drug with actions to raise heart rate. Most commonly encountered drugs are sympathomimetics with actions at β_1 receptors, although antimuscarinic drugs, including atropine or glycopyrrolate, also have positive chronotropic effects.

Index: see Section 2.5.1: Sympathomimetic drugs

Related glossary terms: Adrenaline; Atropine; Ephedrine

Circle breathing system

A circle breathing system (also known as a circle system, or simply a circle) is a breathing system designed to recycle anaesthetic gases, reducing gas usage. The system is composed of two hoses: one to carry gases to the patient from the machine and a separate hose to carry exhaled gases back. Unidirectional valves must be present in each limb to control the direction of flow. The system must also have a means of removing waste CO_2 added to expired gases by the patient, before it can be recycled and returned to the inspiratory limb. CO_2 is removed ('scrubbed') chemically by soda lime, a mixture of calcium and sodium hydroxide.

The system is highly efficient, because inhaled anaesthetic agents are minimally metabolized and therefore are present unchanged in the expired gas. This gas, suitably scrubbed of CO_2, can therefore be returned to the patient to maintain anaesthesia.

Safe use of a circle system depends on gas concentration measurement, as gas concentrations at the airway increasingly differ from the settings at the anaesthetic machine (particularly, settings selected on the vaporizer) as flow rates reduce, because an increasing fraction of the gas present in the inspiratory limb is composed of expired gases that have been recycled.

Index: see Section 1.2.9: Breathing circuits; see Section 1.4.5: Anaesthetic agent monitoring; see Section 1.5: Machine checks; see Chapter 4: Routine induction of general anaesthesia; see Chapter 5: The rapid sequence induction; see Section 7.4: High airway pressures

Related glossary terms: Breathing circuit; Soda lime

Codeine phosphate

Codeine is a naturally occurring opioid (opiate) derived from the opium poppy *Papaver somniferum*. It is a weak opioid agonist and can be used on step 3 of the WHO analgesic ladder.

Much of the clinical effect of codeine depends on metabolism to morphine in the liver. Ten per cent of the UK population lack the enzyme for this transformation and experience little benefit from the drug.

Adult doses are usually 30–60 mg, 4–6-hourly, to a maximum of 240 mg/day.

Index: see Section 2.6.3.1: Codeine phosphate; see Section 3.4.4: Post-operative care

Related glossary terms: Opiate; Opioid; Opioid receptors; ***Papaver somniferum****; WHO analgesic ladder*

Colloids

Colloids are solutions for IV infusion, generally reserved for use in resuscitation. In addition to ions, such as sodium and chloride, they contain protein molecules. The protein component is osmotically active, but cannot diffuse out from plasma, and therefore will tend to retain fluid within the intravascular compartment.

There is little evidence that colloid solutions are more effective in resuscitation than crystalloids. They are both more expensive and potential triggers of anaphylaxis, and many anaesthetists would tend to give only crystalloid solutions under most circumstances.

Example colloid solutions include Gelofusine® (sodium chloride and succinylated gelatine), manufactured by B Braun.

Index: see Section 7.7: Anaphylaxis
Related glossary terms: Crystalloid solutions

Common gas outlet

The CGO is the point on the anaesthetic machine by which each of the components of the FGF (oxygen, air/nitrous oxide, anaesthetic agent) have been added and mixed. It is a single point of connection for a breathing circuit.

Some anaesthetic machines also have an auxiliary CGO fitted to allow for a Mapleson circuit to be connected as well as a circle system. While convenient, this increases the risk of awareness or hypoxia, because, if the selector switch is in the wrong position, no gas will be delivered to the breathing circuit.

Index: see Section 1.2.7: The common gas outlet
Related glossary terms: Fresh gas flow

Controlled drug

A controlled drug is a substance limited by the Misuse of Drugs Act 1971 and Misuse of Drugs Regulations 2001, which place limitations on the manufacture, distribution, and use of certain drugs. Many controlled drugs have useful therapeutic properties, and there are strict rules governing the prescription and handling of controlled drugs.

There are five schedules of controlled drugs:

- **Schedule 1:** drugs with no clinical use and are therefore only legally useable under licence from the Home Office for research
- **Schedule 2:** includes most opioids and cocaine. Prescriptions must include full details, and a written register of stocks must be maintained. Drugs must be secured in double-locked cupboards
- **Schedule 3:** includes some benzodiazepines (midazolam, temazepam, flunitrazepam), barbiturates, and buprenorphine. Requirements are broadly similar to schedule 2, but written registers are generally not required and most schedule 3 drugs can be stored in a general dispensary
- **Schedule 4:** includes other benzodiazepines, except those in schedule 3, anabolic steroids, and some hormonal preparations. Not subject to safe custody requirements
- **Schedule 5:** includes preparations which, by virtue of low strength, are exempt from most controlled drug requirements, other than retention of documentation for 2 years.

Index: see Section 2.6.3: Opioids
Related glossary terms: Fentanyl; Morphine sulfate

Cricoid pressure

Cricoid pressure, or the Sellick manoeuvre, is a technique performed during RSI to occlude the oesophagus. The cricoid cartilage is the only complete cartilaginous ring in the trachea. Pressure applied is therefore transmitted to the oesophagus, compressing it against the body of the C6 vertebrae.

The technique may reduce the risk of aspiration from passive regurgitation, but, if the patient starts to actively vomit, cricoid pressure must be released because of a risk of oesophageal rupture.

Although widely practised in the UK, it is less common in other countries in Europe, and there is little strong evidence to confirm its efficacy.

Index: see Chapter 5: The rapid sequence induction; see Section 7.2: Airway problems at induction

Related glossary terms: Rapid sequence induction

Crystalloid solutions

Crystalloid solutions are simple salt solutions. Examples include saline 0.9% or Hartmann's solution. They are commonly used for both IV fluid maintenance and in resuscitation. They are isotonic, cheap, and non-allergenic. Saline 0.9% contains 150 mmol/L sodium and 150 mmol/L chloride; therefore, 1 L represents almost the entire daily requirement of sodium for a 70 kg person.

Hartmann's solution contains 131 mmol/L sodium, 5 mmol/L potassium, 2 mmol/L calcium, 111 mmol/L chloride, and 29 mmol/L lactate. The lactate is metabolized to bicarbonate in the liver after administration; therefore, the concentrations in Hartmann's solution more closely mirror the ionic composition of plasma.

Index: see Section 7.7: Anaphylaxis

Related glossary terms: Colloids

Cyclo-oxygenase

COX is an enzyme responsible for the generation of prostaglandins, prostacyclin, and thromboxane. The enzyme exists in two isoforms: COX1 and COX2. Both forms of COX metabolize arachidonic acid.

- **COX1** is a constituent enzyme present in all tissues and generates prostaglandins involved in renal blood flow (PgE2, PgI2), platelet function (thromboxane A2), and gastric protection
- **COX2** is an inducible enzyme and is only found in inflamed tissue. COX2 generates proinflammatory prostaglandins.

Broadly, inhibition of COX1 is responsible for many of the side effects of NSAIDs, while COX2 inhibition produces useful clinical effects. Bronchoconstriction is caused by the generation of leukotrienes, an alternative metabolic pathway by which arachidonic acid is metabolized when COX is inhibited.

Index: see Section 2.6.2: Non-steroidal anti-inflammatory drugs

Related glossary terms: Diclofenac; Ibuprofen; Non-steroidal anti-inflammatory drugs

Dantrolene

Dantrolene is a drug that inhibits excitation–contraction coupling in muscle cells by actions on the ryanodine receptor of the sarcoplasmic reticulum. It is used as a specific treatment for patients with MH.

It is given in doses of 2.5 mg/kg, with repeat doses of 1 mg/kg, up to a maximum of 10 mg/kg. The drug is relatively insoluble in water, so drawing it up takes time. During an MH crisis, it may be necessary to allocate a helper to draw up the drug.

Index: see Section 7.11: Malignant hyperthermia

Related glossary terms: Malignant hyperthermia

Dead space

The volume of gas taken in with each breath that is not available for gas exchange is referred to as dead space. In anaesthetic practice, dead space is composed of two components: anatomical and circuit dead space.

- **Anatomical dead space:** this includes the volume contained within the conducting airways (those airways from the lips to the respiratory bronchioles) that do not participate in gas exchange. In a normal adult, the proportion of anatomical dead space is approximately one-third of the tidal volume

- **Circuit dead space:** this represents the volume of gas contained within the circuit between the patient's lips and the FGF. It is functionally equivalent to lengthening the patient's trachea and generally represents the volume of the HME filter, catheter mount, angle-piece, and volume within the airway device itself. Although seldom an issue in adult anaesthesia, it can be a significant factor when anaesthetizing small children and infants.

Index: see Section 1.2.9: Breathing circuits
Related glossary terms: HME filter; Mapleson F; Tidal volume

Depolarizing muscle relaxant

Depolarizing muscle relaxants are agonists at the nicotinic acetylcholine receptor of the neuromuscular junction. They bind to the receptor, activating it and opening the associated ion channel. The drug remains bound to the receptor for longer than acetylcholine, which renders the post-junctional membrane tetanic (i.e. it cannot be further stimulated). This initial depolarization is responsible for the fasciculations seen after administering a dose.

The only depolarizing muscle relaxant in clinical use is suxamethonium.

Depolarizing muscle relaxants are not reversible using neostigmine.

Index: see Section 2.4: Muscle relaxants and reversal agents
Related glossary terms: Neostigmine and glycopyrrolate; Suxamethonium

Desflurane

Desflurane is an inhalational anaesthetic agent with exceptionally quick onset and offset. It is an irritant at light planes of anaesthesia and is unsuitable for inhalational induction. See Table 8.1 for its properties.

Index: see Section 1.2.6: Anaesthetic vaporizers; see Section 1.5: Machine checks; see Section 2.3: Inhalational anaesthetic agents
Related glossary terms: Anaesthetic agent potency; Anaesthetic agent solubility

Dexamethasone

Dexamethasone is a powerful synthetic glucocorticoid, with potency seven times that of prednisolone and 27 times that of cortisol.

It is frequently used in anaesthesia for its antiemetic properties where it is given as a single dose of 8 mg at induction.

Index: see Section 2.7.1.1: Dexamethasone; see Chapter 4: Routine induction of general anaesthesia; see Chapter 5: The rapid sequence induction

Diclofenac

Diclofenac is an NSAID derived from phenylacetic acid. Non-steroidal drugs form step 2 of the WHO analgesic ladder.

Adult oral doses are usually 50 mg, 8-hourly, to a maximum of 150 mg/day.

Index: see Section 2.6.2.2: Diclofenac; see Section 3.4.4: Post-operative care

Table 8.1 Properties of desflurane

	Colour code	MAC	Boiling point	Molecular weight	Blood:gas partition coefficient
Sevoflurane	Yellow	2.00	58.5°C	200.1	0.70
Isoflurane	Purple	1.10	48.5°C	184.5	1.40
Desflurane	**Blue**	**6.35**	**22.8°C**	**168.0**	**0.45**

Related glossary terms: Cyclo-oxygenase; Ibuprofen; Non-steroidal anti-inflammatory drugs; WHO analgesic ladder

Difficult airway

Although no standard definition exists, a difficult airway is one in which an anaesthetist, with a reasonable degree of skill and experience, would find it difficult to face mask-ventilate a patient, perform tracheal intubation, or both.

Note that the term difficult airway is not synonymous with difficult intubation. Patients that are difficult to face mask ventilate may in fact be easy to intubate (e.g. edentulous patients). Some patients that are difficult to intubate may be easy to mask ventilate. Patients that are both difficult to mask ventilate and intubate present particular hazards for the anaesthetist.

Index: see Section 1.5: Machine checks; see Section 3.2.2: Airway assessment; see Section 7.2: Airway problems at induction; see Section 7.5: Airway problems at extubation

Related glossary terms: Rapid sequence induction

Difficult Airway Society

The DAS is a group of anaesthetists, founded in 1995 to promote training and management of difficult airway situations in anaesthesia and critical care. The Society has produced a number of guidelines to assist in the management of difficult intubation and other critical airway situations.

Index: see Section 3.2.2: Airway assessment; see Section 3.4: Planning a general anaesthetic; see Section 7.2: Airway problems at induction

Related glossary terms: Difficult airway; Difficult intubation; Failed intubation drill

Difficult intubation

A difficult intubation is loosely defined as an intubation that a reasonably skilled and experienced anaesthetist has difficulty performing. Broadly, a Cormack and Lehane grade III or IV view at direct laryngoscopy implies difficulty.

Difficulty may be caused by anatomical factors, pathology, or by poor patient positioning prior to induction. Commonly, combinations of all three factors complicate clinical practice.

Every attempt should be made to identify patients at risk of difficult intubation prior to theatre so that adequate preparations can be made to reduce risk, including alternative intubation strategies.

The UK DAS has produced a series of guidelines to assist the dealing with failed intubations.

The term is distinct from 'difficult airway', which also encompasses difficult face mask ventilation, although, in clinical practice, the terms are often used interchangeably.

Index: see Section 3.2.2: Airway assessment; see Section 7.2: Airway problems at induction; see Section 7.5: Airway problems at extubation

Related glossary terms: Difficult airway; Difficult Airway Society; Failed intubation drill

EMLA®

EMLA® cream, or Eutectic Mixture of Local Anaesthetic, is a topical anaesthetic frequently used before cannulation, especially in children. It contains a mixture of 2.5% lidocaine and 2.5% prilocaine—by combining the two agents in equal proportions, the melting point of the mixture is lower than the melting point of the two constituents alone. Essentially, this means that it forms a gel that can be easily applied, without requiring any additional solvents.

It takes around 60 min to work and needs to be covered with an occlusive dressing after application. Anaesthesia lasts for up to 2 h after removing the dressing.

Index: see Section 2.8: Local anaesthetics

Related glossary terms: Ametop®; Lidocaine; Prilocaine

Enantiomers

An enantiomer is a form of chemical isomer. Isomers are molecules that share the same chemical formula, but the molecule is of a different shape.

Enantiomers are mirror images of each other but are not superimposable. Enantiomers are labelled as either R or S forms of the molecule, based on the arrangement of molecular subgroups around the chiral carbon or nitrogen atom.

Many drugs in clinical use are enantiomers, but some of the more commonly encountered in anaesthetic practice include bupivacaine, isoflurane, desflurane, atropine, and ketamine.

A racemic mixture is one in which both enantiomers are present in equal proportions.

Index: see Section 2.8.2: Bupivacaine

Related glossary terms: Atropine; Bupivacaine; Desflurane; Isoflurane; Racemic mixture

End-tidal carbon dioxide

End-tidal CO_2 concentration, or E_tCO_2, is the concentration of CO_2 present at the end of expiration of a normal tidal-volume breath. This reflects the concentration of CO_2 in the blood, and the value reflects the adequacy of ventilation.

Index: see Section 1.3.4: Tracheal tubes; see Section 1.4.4: End-tidal capnography; see Chapter 4: Routine induction of general anaesthesia; see Chapter 5: The rapid sequence induction

Related glossary terms: Minute volume; Tidal volume

Ephedrine

Ephedrine is a sympathomimetic, with mixed α- and β-effects, which can be used in the treatment of hypotension. It causes peripheral vasoconstriction, increased heart rate (positive chronotropy), and increased contractility (positive inotropy).

Effects are mediated by the potentiation of noradrenaline from sympathetic nerve terminals, so its use is complicated by tachyphylaxis as noradrenaline stocks are depleted.

Index: see Section 2.5.1.1: Ephedrine; see Section 3.4: Planning a general anaesthetic; see Chapter 4: Routine induction of general anaesthesia; see Chapter 5: The rapid sequence induction

Related glossary terms: Chronotrope; Inotrope; Tachyphylaxis

Epidural anaesthesia

Epidural anaesthesia involves the placement of a plastic catheter into the epidural space around the spine. Most commonly sited in the lumbar region to provide analgesia or anaesthesia in obstetric practice, they can also be used to provide anaesthesia for orthopaedic surgery and, if placed in the thoracic region, can provide good-quality pain relief after major abdominal operations.

Epidural drug mixtures usually contain an LA, often lidocaine or bupivacaine, and a lipid-soluble opioid such as fentanyl or diamorphine. Doses for epidural analgesia are lower than those used to achieve anaesthesia.

Epidural anaesthesia takes longer to reach peak effect compared to spinal anaesthetics, but has the advantage that adding additional doses via the catheter can prolong their effect beyond that seen with 'spinals'.

Index: see Chapter 6: Central neuraxial blockade

Related glossary terms: Bupivacaine; Fentanyl; Lidocaine; Spinal anaesthesia

Extrapyramidal side effects

Extrapyramidal side effects arise from central antagonism of dopaminergic receptors. A spectrum of clinical conditions is observed:

- **Acute dystonic reactions:** abnormal muscular spasms, including torticollis and oculogyric crisis
- **Akathisia:** a subjective feeling of motor restlessness
- **Pseudoparkinsonism:** features are similar to Parkinson's disease, characterized by rigidity and bradykinesia
- **Tardive dyskinesia:** tardive dyskinesia is associated with involuntary and asymmetric movements of muscle groups. It is a condition seen after chronic use of drugs affecting

dopaminergic transmission, typically anti-psychotic medications in the context of long-term psychotic illness.

Index: see Section 2.7.3.1: Metoclopramide
Related glossary terms: Metoclopramide

Failed intubation drill

A failed intubation drill is a rehearsed sequence of actions to be taken in the event that direct laryngoscopy and tracheal intubation prove difficult or impossible. The most widely accepted guidelines in UK practice were published by DAS in 2007.

It is good practice for every anaesthetist to mentally rehearse this drill before every intubation.

Index: see Section 1.3: Airway management; see Section 7.2: Airway problems at induction
Related glossary terms: Difficult airway; Difficult Airway Society; Difficult intubation

Fentanyl

Fentanyl is a synthetic opioid with approximately ten times the potency of morphine. It is often administered during anaesthesia where it is given in IV boluses of 1 microgram/kg. It has faster onset than morphine and a shorter duration of action. Given prior to induction, it can suppress the sympathetic response to laryngoscopy, which can be valuable in some clinical situations.

Fentanyl can also be given by continuous infusion for sedation purposes, be used in PCA regimens, and incorporated into mixtures for spinal or epidural anaesthesia.

Index: see Section 2.6.3.2: Fentanyl; see Section 3.4: Planning a general anaesthetic; see Chapter 4: Routine induction of general anaesthesia; see Chapter 5: The rapid sequence induction; see Chapter 6: Central neuraxial blockade
Related glossary terms: Epidural anaesthesia; Opioid; Opioid receptors; Spinal anaesthesia

F_iO_2

F_iO_2 is the oxygen concentration of inspired gas, expressed as a decimal of 1. The F_iO_2 when breathing atmospheric air (21% oxygen) would equal 0.21, whereas breathing 100% oxygen would imply an F_iO_2 of 1.0.

Index: see Section 3.4: Planning a general anaesthetic

Flowmeter

A flowmeter is a device for measuring gas flow. They are present in anaesthetic machines (where they may be physical or electronic) and also on wall oxygen outlets or gas cylinders.

Physical flowmeters must be in the upright position to be read correctly.

Flowmeters are calibrated to specific gases, as they depend on characteristics such as density and viscosity. A bobbin is suspended within the gas stream to enable the gas flow to be read against a calibrated scale. The scale is usually given in L/min on gas cylinders and wall outlets. On an anaesthetic machine, two flowmeters may be connected in series for each gas, with the first flowmeter calibrated in mL/min and the second in L/min.

Index: see Section 1.2.5: The flowmeter; see Section 1.5: Machine checks; see Chapter 4: Routine induction of general anaesthesia; see Chapter 5: The rapid sequence induction; see Section 7.9: Adult advanced life support

Fresh gas flow

FGF refers to the stream of gas delivered by the CGO of the anaesthetic machine. By the time gas has reached the CGO, it has been through the flowmeters and back-bar. At this point, it will contain oxygen, air or nitrous oxide, and a volatile anaesthetic agent (depending on the settings chosen by the anaesthetist).

The required FGF rate depends on the breathing circuit used; in a circle system, the FGF rate can theoretically be as low as 250 mL/min (essentially supplying only the patient's metabolic

oxygen requirements), although, in practice, higher flow rates are usually used to compensate for small leaks in the system. Flow rates must be much higher when using Mapleson circuits to prevent rebreathing.
Index: see Section 1.2.5: The flowmeter; see Section 1.2.9: Breathing circuits; see Section 1.4.4: End-tidal capnography
Related glossary terms: Circle breathing system; Common gas outlet; Mapleson classification; Rebreathing

Gauge pressure

Gauge pressure is a pressure measurement relative to atmospheric pressure. An empty gas cylinder would have a gauge pressure of 0 kPa. Gauge pressure can be thought of as absolute pressure minus atmospheric pressure. Most measurements in clinical practice are gauge pressures.
Index: see Section 1.2.3: Pressure gauges
Related glossary terms: Absolute pressure; Pascal

Heat sink

A heat sink is a component in a system with a high specific heat capacity. It is used in many electrical systems, as well as anaesthetic vaporizers, as a means of absorbing and dissipating heat. The presence of a heat sink thereby helps to maintain a more constant temperature within the system.

In an anaesthetic vaporizer, the heat sink is usually composed of a large piece of copper.
Index: see Section 1.2.6: Anaesthetic vaporizers

Heavy bupivacaine

Heavy bupivacaine is a specific preparation of the LA agent bupivacaine, used for spinal anaesthesia.

The mixture contains 0.5% (5 mg/mL) bupivacaine, with 8% (80 mg/mL) glucose. The addition of glucose raises the specific gravity of the solution, making it denser than CSF. This affords the benefit of making the mixture move predictably in CSF, allowing the anaesthetist to control its spread by careful positioning of the patient.
Index: see Section 2.8.2: Bupivacaine; see Chapter 6: Central neuraxial blockade
Related glossary terms: Bupivacaine; Spinal anaesthesia

HME filter

The HME is a filter placed in the breathing circuit close to the patient's airway. It consists of a fine mesh of a hygroscopic material that causes moisture from the patient's lungs to condense upon it during expiration and evaporate again into the inspired gas. This has the double benefit of maintaining warmth and humidity on the patient side of the filter whilst simultaneously keeping the machine side dry and free from contamination.
Index: see Section 7.3: Loss of capnography waveform

Hofmann elimination

Hofmann elimination, first described by August Wilhelm von Hofmann, is the degradation of a quaternary amine (like atracurium) to yield an alkene and a tertiary amine. The process is spontaneous and is more rapid at higher temperatures.
Index: see Section 2.4.1.1: Atracurium
Related glossary terms: Atracurium

Hudson mask

A variable performance face mask used for delivery of oxygen therapy. The F_iO_2 delivered depends on the patient's respiratory effort, respiratory rate, and the flow rate of the attached oxygen.

When connected to a reservoir bag (commonly, but incorrectly, referred to as a non-rebreathe bag), the delivered F_iO_2 rises but again is dependent on the patient's effort and respiratory rate.

If a venturi is connected, the device delivers a known concentration of oxygen, specified on the venturi device. A venturi is described as a fixed-performance device, because the F_iO_2 delivered is not affected by patient factors.

Index: see Section 7.5: Airway problems at extubation

Human factors

'Human factors' is a complex field that studies the properties of human–human and human–machine interaction. It combines elements of psychology, engineering, behavioural science, and anthropometry.

Human factors is concerned with the systems that people work within and how those systems can be designed to minimize risk. Many of the elements are described by 'non-technical skills', including effective communication, team working, and situational awareness.

High-stakes industries, notably nuclear power and aviation, have shown great interest in human factors for several decades, but it has only been relatively recently that the medical profession has investigated its implications. Anaesthesia has been at the forefront of medical human factors.

The death of Elaine Bromiley on 29 March 2005 was a significant event in medical human factors training (see Section 7.1).

Index: see Section 3.5: Communication in theatre; see Section 7.2: Airway problems at induction; see Section 7.9.3: Human factors in resuscitation

I:E ratio

I:E ratio, or the ratio of inspiratory to expiratory time, is one of the settings that can be controlled during artificial ventilation. A normal I:E ratio is 1:2; therefore, expiration takes twice as long as inspiration.

It is only occasionally that the anaesthetist is required to change I:E ratio in theatre anaesthesia. By reducing I:E ratio to 1:1.5, proportionally more time is available for inspiration; therefore, breaths can be delivered more slowly and with lower inspiratory pressures. I:E ratios of 1:1 are used in ICU, but rarely in theatre, as the reduction in expiratory time increases the risk of incomplete expiration, causing gas to be trapped within the lungs.

Index: see Section 1.2.10: The ventilator; see Section 7.4: High airway pressures

Ibuprofen

Ibuprofen is an NSAID derived from propanoic acid. Ibuprofen is thought to have the lowest rate of side effects of all non-steroidal drugs but is only available as an oral preparation in the UK.

Non-steroidal drugs form step 2 of the WHO analgesic ladder. Usual adult doses are 400 mg, 4–6-hourly, to a maximum of 2.4 g/day.

Index: see Section 2.6.2.1: Ibuprofen; see Section 3.4.4: Post-operative care

Related glossary terms: Cyclo-oxygenase; Diclofenac; WHO analgesic ladder

Inhalational induction

Inhalational induction (also known as gas induction) is a method of inducing general anaesthesia without recourse to IV agents.

It is most commonly achieved using sevoflurane, with or without nitrous oxide. It is commonly practised in children who may be overly upset by IV cannulation. Standard monitoring requirements still apply.

It is occasionally practised in adults and in some difficult airway situations, under the supervision of senior anaesthetists.

Index: see Section 2.3.1: Sevoflurane
Related glossary terms: Second gas effect; Sevoflurane

Inotrope

Technically, an inotrope is a drug with positive inotropic properties (i.e. increases myocardial contractility), although the term is often used in day-to-day practice to refer to any potent drug used to support blood pressure.

Most inotropic drugs are direct-acting β_1 agonists that act on the heart to increase stroke volume. Commonly used agents include adrenaline, noradrenaline, dopamine, and isoprenaline. Specific β_2 agonists, like salbutamol, would not be described as inotropes. Many inotropes are also positive chronotropes.

Index: see Section 2.5.1.1: Ephedrine; see Section 2.5.1.3: Adrenaline; see Section 3.4: Planning a general anaesthetic

Isoflurane

Isoflurane is an inhalational anaesthetic agent with higher potency, but slower onset and offset, when compared with sevoflurane or desflurane. It is pungent and can irritate the airways at light planes of anaesthesia. Isoflurane is unsuitable for inhalational induction. See Table 8.2 for its properties.

Index: see Section 1.2.6: Anaesthetic vaporizers; see Section 2.3.2: Isoflurane; see Section 3.4: Planning a general anaesthetic; see Chapter 4: Routine induction of general anaesthesia; see Chapter 5: The rapid sequence induction; see Section 7.4: High airway pressures

Related glossary terms: Anaesthetic agent potency; Anaesthetic agent solubility

Jet ventilator

A jet ventilator is a high-pressure oxygen device, operating between 100 and 400 kPa. It requires connection to a high-pressure supply via a Schrader valve. Although occasionally used electively in shared airway surgery (e.g. ENT microlaryngoscopy), it has an important role in 'can't intubate–can't ventilate' scenarios as an airway rescue technique.

The device is connected via a Luer lock to a needle cricothyroidotomy cannula and short bursts of oxygen applied. This can maintain oxygenation of the patient, while steps are taken to achieve definitive management of the airway. Patients can be oxygenated for 30 min or more using this technique, although its use is limited by poor elimination of CO_2.

When using a jet ventilator, it is not possible to exhale through the jet ventilator or cannula, so some anatomical airway must be maintained.

Index: see Section 7.2: Airway problems at induction
Related glossary terms: Failed intubation drill; Schrader valve

Laryngospasm

Laryngospasm is the reflex closure of the vocal cords, occluding the airway. It is a normal protective response to upper airway stimulation that protects the trachea from soiling but, as it causes airway occlusion, it can lead to hypoxia if uncontrolled.

Table 8.2 Properties of isoflurane

	Colour code	MAC	Boiling point	Molecular weight	Blood:gas partition coefficient
Sevoflurane	Yellow	2.00	58.5°C	200.1	0.70
Isoflurane	**Purple**	**1.10**	**48.5°C**	**184.5**	**1.40**
Desflurane	Blue	6.35	22.8°C	168.0	0.45

Treatment includes PEEP, deepening anaesthesia, or small doses of suxamethonium.
Index: see Section 2.3: Inhalational anaesthetic agents; see Section 2.4.2.1: Suxamethonium; see Section 3.4: Planning a general anaesthetic; see Section 7.3: Loss of capnography waveform; see Section 7.5: Airway problems at extubation
Related glossary terms: PEEP; Suxamethonium

Lidocaine

Lidocaine is a commonly used LA agent that can be used for local infiltration, peripheral nerve blockade, or epidural anaesthesia. It has a quicker onset, but shorter duration of action, than bupivacaine. Historically, it was also used as an anti-arrhythmic in the treatment of ventricular arrhythmias, although this role has been largely supplanted by more modern agents.

It is usually presented as 1% or 2% solutions, with or without 1:200 000 adrenaline. It is also available mixed with prilocaine (as EMLA® cream) for topical anaesthesia and as a 10% oral spray.

The maximum dose is 3 mg/kg, although, when given with adrenaline up to 7 mg/kg can be administered.
Index: see Section 2.8.1: Lidocaine; see Chapter 6: Central neuraxial blockade; see Section 7.8: Local anaesthetic toxicity; see Section 7.10.1: Tachycardia
Related glossary terms: Bupivacaine; EMLA®; Local anaesthetics; Prilocaine

Local anaesthetics

An LA is a drug that reversibly inhibits transmission in sensory nerves. They have a role in topical anaesthesia, local infiltration of wounds, peripheral nerve blocks, and central neuraxial blocks.

LAs block fast sodium channels, inhibiting propagation of action potentials along the nerve. This effect is not specific to sensory nerves; blockade of sodium channels in myocytes and in the CNS is responsible for potentially hazardous toxic effects.
Index: see Section 2.8: Local anaesthetics; see Chapter 6: Central neuraxial blockade; see Section 7.8: Local anaesthetic toxicity
Related glossary terms: Bupivacaine; Epidural anaesthesia; Lidocaine; Spinal anaesthesia

Malignant hyperthermia

Malignant hyperthermia (also known as malignant hyperpyrexia or MH) is an autosomal dominant abnormality of skeletal muscle calcium channels that results in a hypermetabolic state when exposed to certain trigger agents. All volatile anaesthetic agents and suxamethonium are trigger agents for MH.

The condition affects 1:200 000 in the UK and is characterized by excessive calcium release from the sarcoplasmic reticulum, causing overactivity of muscular contraction. This generates CO_2, heat, and lactate. The condition can be fatal, if not promptly treated.

Clinical features include masseter spasm, unexplained tachycardia, and hypercapnia.

Hyperthermia is a late sign.

Treatment is with dantrolene, aggressive cooling, and correction of biochemical abnormalities.
Index: see Section 2.4.2.1: Suxamethonium; see Section 3.2.1: The anaesthetic history; see Section 7.11: Malignant hyperthermia
Related glossary terms: Desflurane; Isoflurane; Sevoflurane; Suxamethonium

Mapleson C

The Mapleson C system, also called a Waters bag, is a compact anaesthetic circuit. It is inefficient in terms of gas usage, limiting its use in routine anaesthesia; however, it has a role in resuscitation and patient transfer. It is broadly similar to a bag–valve–mask system, like an Ambu-bag™, although with two key differences: it has an APL valve, which permits the user to set the airway pressure, and the bag is not self-inflating. The system must therefore be connected to a gas supply.

The system is functionally similar to a Mapleson D circuit, although it lacks a length of hose. It consists of a reservoir bag in the inspiratory limb of the circuit, with fresh gas added close to the reservoir bag. The exhaust valve is between the fresh gas input and the patient's airway.

Index: see Section 1.2.9: Breathing circuits

Related glossary terms: Breathing circuit; Mapleson C; Mapleson classification; Mapleson D; Mapleson F; Rebreathing

Mapleson classification

William W Mapleson was a Cardiff-based physicist who described a system of classifying anaesthetic circuits, based on the relative positions of the APL (exhaust) valve, the fresh gas input, and the reservoir bag. There are six circuits described in the system, denoted by letters A to F. Only circuits C, D, and F are in common clinical use.

Index: see Section 1.2.9.1: Rebreathing systems

Related glossary terms: Breathing circuit; Mapleson C; Mapleson classification; Mapleson D; Mapleson F; Rebreathing

Mapleson D

The Mapleson D circuit, often referred to as a Bain circuit, is commonly used in the anaesthetic room, as it is more compact and technically simpler than a circle system. It is less efficient in terms of gas consumption than a circle, so it is less commonly used for prolonged anaesthesia in theatre.

The system delivers fresh gas near the patient end, with an exhaust valve and a reservoir bag in the expiratory limb.

The system requires fresh gas flows of 2–4 times the patient's minute volume to prevent rebreathing.

Index: see Section 1.2.9: Breathing circuits; see Section 1.5: Machine checks

Related glossary terms: Breathing circuit; Circle breathing system; Mapleson C; Mapleson classification; Mapleson F; Rebreathing

Mapleson F

The Mapleson F system is the Jackson–Rees modification of the Ayre's T-piece (Mapleson E) and is commonly referred to as a 'T-piece'.

The system is composed of a length of corrugated hose ending in a standard connector for the airway or face mask. At the other end of the hose is an open-ended reservoir bag. Fresh gas is introduced at the patient end, near the airway connector.

The system has low dead space and, since it has no valves, it is of very low resistance. This makes it suitable for paediatric use. Flow rates of 2–3 times the minute volume are generally required to prevent rebreathing.

Index: see Section 1.2.9: Breathing circuits

Related glossary terms: Breathing circuit; Mapleson C; Mapleson classification; Mapleson D; Rebreathing

Metaraminol

Metaraminol is a synthetic amine with predominantly α_1 adrenergic effects, although it retains some β-effects too. It is used in the treatment of hypotension, acting to cause peripheral vasoconstriction. Reflex bradycardia can be seen in response to the increase in systemic vascular resistance.

Index: see Section 2.5.1.2: Metaraminol; see Section 3.4: Planning a general anaesthetic; see Chapter 4: Routine induction of general anaesthesia; see Chapter 5: The rapid sequence induction

Related glossary terms: Vasopressor

Metoclopramide

Metoclopramide is an antiemetic and prokinetic drug which acts predominantly through competitive antagonism of D_2 receptors in the CTZ, although it also has some activity at 5-HT_3 receptors.

It is available for oral, IV, or IM use. Extrapyramidal side effects can complicate the use of metoclopramide.

Index: see Section 2.7.3.1: Metoclopramide

Related glossary terms: Chemoreceptor trigger zone; Extrapyramidal side effects

Minimum alveolar concentration

MAC is the concentration of inhaled anaesthetic agent required to prevent movement to a defined surgical stimulus in 50% of non-premedicated patients. MAC is generally used as a means of determining potency of an anaesthetic agent and is used clinically to guide administration of volatiles. Keeping end-tidal agent concentrations above 1 MAC reduces awareness risk. See Table 8.3 for the MAC values of commonly used anaesthetics.

MAC varies with age, tending to be higher in children, and can be affected by conditions such as hyperthyroidism. Sedative drugs, including benzodiazepines and opioids, reduce MAC, as does the inhaled agent nitrous oxide. MAC can be increased by stimulant drugs, including cocaine and adrenaline.

Index: see Section 1.4.5: Anaesthetic agent monitoring; see Section 2.3: Inhalational anaesthetic agents; see Section 3.4: Planning a general anaesthetic; see Chapter 4: Routine induction of general anaesthesia; see Chapter 5: The rapid sequence induction

Minute volume

Minute volume is the volume of gas displaced by respiratory effort over 1 min. It is calculated by multiplying tidal volume by respiratory rate. Minute volume is usually in the range of 5–6 L/min in an average sized adult.

E_tCO_2 concentration is inversely related to minute volume, so E_tCO_2 can be used as an estimate of the adequacy of ventilation.

Index: see Section 1.2.10: The ventilator; see Section 1.4.4: End-tidal capnography

Related glossary terms: End-tidal carbon dioxide; Tidal volume

Mivacurium

Mivacurium is a non-depolarizing muscle relaxant, structurally related to atracurium. It is infrequently used due to low potency and short duration of action. It is unusual amongst non-depolarizing relaxants, since it is broken down by plasma cholinesterases (like suxamethonium) so is not reversible with neostigmine. The duration of action of mivacurium is also prolonged in suxamethonium apnoea, unlike the other non-depolarizing agents.

Index: see Section 7.6: Suxamethonium apnoea

Related glossary terms: Atracurium; Suxamethonium; Suxamethonium apnoea

Morphine sulfate

Morphine is a naturally occurring alkaloid derived from the opium poppy *Papaver somniferum*.

Table 8.3 MAC values for commonly used anaesthetics

Agent	MAC in air
Sevoflurane	2.00
Isoflurane	1.10
Desflurane	6.35

It is the prototypical opioid drug against which others are compared. It acts via opioid receptors to cause analgesia, sedation, respiratory depression, miosis, and constipation.

Dependence and tolerance develop with prolonged use, but this is seldom an issue in the short-term treatment of acute pain.

Morphine has an important role in the treatment of pain, at WHO analgesic ladder step 4, and is commonly used in the perioperative period. It is usually given towards the end of major surgery (in a dose of 0.1 mg/kg) or as rescue analgesia in recovery.

Index: see Section 2.6.3.3: Morphine sulfate

Related glossary terms: Opiate; Opioid; Opioid receptors; ***Papaver somniferum****; Rescue analgesia; WHO analgesic ladder*

Muscarinic acetylcholine receptor

Muscarinic acetylcholine receptors are found in the central and autonomic nervous systems. They are G-protein-linked receptors and mediate transmission of parasympathetic signals in the autonomic system. Activation causes clinical effects including bradycardia and bronchoconstriction.

Atropine and glycopyrrolate both act to inhibit transmission at muscarinic receptors.

Index: see Section 2.4: Muscle relaxants and reversal agents; see Section 2.5.2: Anticholinergic drugs

Related glossary terms: Atropine; Nicotinic acetylcholine receptor

NCEPOD

NCEPOD is a national UK project originally set up to review surgical and anaesthetic care. Originally termed the National Confidential Enquiry into Perioperative Death, it has now expanded to cover all medical specialties.

NCEPOD has produced a number of reports and guidelines relevant to perioperative care.

Index: see Section 3.2.5: NCEPOD grading

Neostigmine and glycopyrrolate

Neostigmine and glycopyrrolate are often presented as a premixed solution of both drugs and is used in the reversal of non-depolarizing neuromuscular blockade.

The neostigmine component inhibits acetylcholinesterase, raising the concentration of acetylcholine at the neuromuscular junction (nicotinic receptors) and throughout the parasympathetic nervous system (muscarinic receptors). This increase in acetylcholine can then compete better for receptor sites occupied by muscle relaxants such as atracurium.

The addition of glycopyrrolate, an antimuscarinic, avoids excessive parasympathetic activation that could result in effects such as bradycardia and bronchoconstriction.

Index: see Section 2.4.3.1: Neostigmine and glycopyrrolate; see Section 3.4: Planning a general anaesthetic; see Section 7.2: Airway problems at induction; see Section 7.5: Airway problems at extubation

Related glossary terms: Atracurium; Muscarinic acetylcholine receptor; Nicotinic acetylcholine receptor; Non-depolarizing muscle relaxant

Nicotinic acetylcholine receptor

The nicotinic acetylcholine receptor is found at the neuromuscular junction. The receptor is linked to an ion channel, and two forms are recognized: one in the autonomic nervous system and the other at the neuromuscular junction.

Non-depolarizing agents, including atracurium, block receptors found at the neuromuscular junction. Suxamethonium activates the receptor but prevents further transmission by taking a long time to dissociate from it, rendering the post-junctional membrane tetanic.

Index: see Section 2.4: Muscle relaxants and reversal agents; see Section 2.5.2: Anticholinergic drugs

Related glossary terms: Atracurium; Non-depolarizing muscle relaxant; Rocuronium; Suxamethonium; Vecuronium

Non-depolarizing muscle relaxant

Non-depolarizing muscle relaxants are a group of neuromuscular blockers that include benzylisoquinolinium drugs (such as atracurium) and aminosteroids (vecuronium and rocuronium).

The drugs are competitive antagonists at the muscarinic acetylcholine receptor of the neuromuscular junction. They bind to the receptors, occupying it without activating it (in pharmacological terms, they have an intrinsic activity of 0) and therefore do not cause depolarization of post-junctional membrane.

Index: see Section 2.4: Muscle relaxants and reversal agents
Related glossary terms: Atracurium; Neostigmine and glycopyrrolate; Rocuronium; Vecuronium

Non-interchangeable screw thread

NISTs refer to the threaded attachments on pipelines connected to the back of the anaesthetic machine. The screw thread on each hose is gas-specific, so it should not be possible to accidentally screw a pipeline into the wrong connector.

Index: see Section 1.2.1: Piped medical gases

Non-rebreathing circuit

Non-rebreathing circuit is another means of describing a circle system. Although rebreathing does not occur at low FGF rates (as it would with a Mapleson system), it should be noted that rebreathing is still possible if the soda lime canister is depleted.

Index: see Section 1.2.9.2: Circle systems
Related glossary terms: Breathing circuit; Circle breathing system; Mapleson classification; Rebreathing; Soda lime

Non-steroidal anti-inflammatory drugs

NSAIDs are a class of drugs that act by inhibition of the COX enzyme. NSAIDs have useful analgesic, antipyretic, and anti-inflammatory properties and are widely used post-operatively as step 2 on the WHO analgesic ladder.

Caution must be exercised in certain patient groups, as NSAIDs are associated with cardiac events, bleeding (especially from the GI tract), peptic ulceration, renal failure, and bronchoconstriction.

Index: see Section 2.6.2: Non-steroidal anti-inflammatory drugs; see Section 3.2.1: The anaesthetic history; see Section 3.4.4: Post-operative care
Related glossary terms: Cyclo-oxygenase; Diclofenac; Ibuprofen; WHO analgesic ladder

Ondansetron

Ondansetron is an antiemetic drug that acts via antagonism of serotonergic (5-HT_3) receptors in the chemical trigger zone.

Side effects are rare, and the drug is commonly used in both adult and paediatric practice. Usual adult doses are 4 mg, 8-hourly, to a maximum of 12 mg/day. It is generally used for up to 24 h post-operatively.

Index: see Section 2.7.4.1: Ondansetron
Related glossary terms: Chemoreceptor trigger zone

Opiate

Opiate is a term that specifically refers to naturally occurring substances with morphine-type properties derived from the *Papaver somniferum* poppy. The only commonly used opiates are morphine and codeine.

Index: see Section 2.6.3: Opioids
Related glossary terms: Codeine phosphate; Morphine sulfate; Opioid; Papaver somniferum

Opioid

Opioid is a term that refers to both naturally occurring and synthetic agonists at the μ family of receptors. Morphine is the prototypical opioid receptor agonist against which other opioids are compared. Morphine and codeine are naturally occurring, while drugs such as fentanyl or remifentanil are synthetic.

Index: see Section 2.6.3: Opioids; see Section 2.7: Antiemetics; see Section 3.2.1: The anaesthetic history; see Section 3.4: Planning a general anaesthetic; see Chapter 4: Routine induction of general anaesthesia; see Chapter 5: The rapid sequence induction

Related glossary terms: Codeine phosphate; Fentanyl; Morphine sulfate; Opiate; Opioid; Opioid receptors; Remifentanil

Opioid receptors

Opioid receptors are a family of receptors distributed throughout the CNS, spinal cord, and GI tract, responsible for the clinical effects of morphine and related drugs.

There are three receptor types: delta (δ), kappa (κ), and mu (μ) (see Table 8.4).

Index: see Section 2.6.3: Opioids

Papaver somniferum

Papaver somniferum is the opium poppy from which naturally occurring opioid drugs (opiates) are derived.

Opium is the latex harvested from seedpods and yields morphine, oripavine, codeine, and thebaine. Neither thebaine nor oripavine have clinically useful properties.

Index: see Section 2.6.3: Opioids

Related glossary terms: Codeine phosphate; Morphine sulfate; Opiate

Paracetamol

Paracetamol is one of the most commonly prescribed analgesics in the world. Its mechanism of action is unclear but is thought to act on prostaglandin synthesis in the CNS.

Side effects are rare, but overdose (accidental or iatrogenic) risks severe hepatotoxicity.

Paracetamol forms step 1 of the WHO analgesic ladder. Usual adult doses are 1 g, 4–6-hourly, to a maximum of 4 g/day.

Index: see Section 2.6.1: Paracetamol; see Section 3.4.4: Post-operative care

Related glossary terms: WHO analgesic ladder

Pascal

The SI unit of pressure, defined as the pressure exerted by a 1 kg mass acting across a surface area of 1 m. This is a very small pressure, so pressure is more usually described in kilopascal (x 10^3 Pa) in anaesthetic practice. Atmospheric pressure is commonly assumed to be approximately 100 kPa.

The unit is named after French physicist Blaise Pascal.

Index: see Section 1.2.1: Piped medical gases; see Section 1.5: Machine checks

Related glossary terms: SI unit

Table 8.4 Opioid receptors

Receptor	Subtypes	Effect
δ	δ_1, δ_2	Analgesia, respiratory depression, dependence
κ	$\kappa_1, \kappa_2, \kappa_3$	Analgesia, sedation, miosis, dysphoria, inhibition of antidiuretic hormone release
μ	μ_1, μ_2, μ_3	μ1: analgesia, dependence μ2: respiratory depression, miosis, euphoria, reduced GI motility

PEEP

PEEP is a supra-atmospheric pressure applied to the lungs at the end of expiration. It can be intrinsic (applied by incomplete expiration which may occur in hyperventilation or the progressive gas trapping seen in asthma) or extrinsic (applied by a ventilator).

Although the application of PEEP increases mean airway pressures, it can be useful in improving hypoxaemia by reducing end-expiratory alveolar collapse and by increasing functional residual capacity (FRC).

The application of PEEP, and therefore the increased intrathoracic pressure, can reduce venous return and increase ICP.

Index: see Section 7.4: High airway pressures; see Section 7.5.3: Laryngospasm

Pin-index system

The pin-index system is a method of reducing the possibility of mounting a cylinder incorrectly on an anaesthetic machine. A series of pins are mounted underneath the gas inlet on the anaesthetic machine that match with holes machined into the cylinder yoke.

Each gas has specific pin positions, so it should not be possible to create a gas-tight seal if the wrong cylinder is connected.

Pin positions are defined by International (ISO) and European (CEN) standards EN ISO 407: Small medical gas cylinders—pin-index yoke-type valve connections.

Commonly used cylinders use the following pin positions (see Fig 8.2):

- Oxygen: 2, 5
- Nitrous oxide: 3, 5
- Air: 1, 5.

Index: see Section 1.2.2: Gas cylinders

Prilocaine

Prilocaine is a short-acting LA agent. It can be used for short-duration peripheral nerve blocks but is perhaps more commonly encountered mixed with lidocaine in EMLA® cream.

Maximum doses are 6 mg/kg (without adrenaline) and 9 mg/kg when mixed with 1:200 000 adrenaline.

Index: see Section 2.8.1: Lidocaine
Related glossary terms: EMLA®; Lidocaine

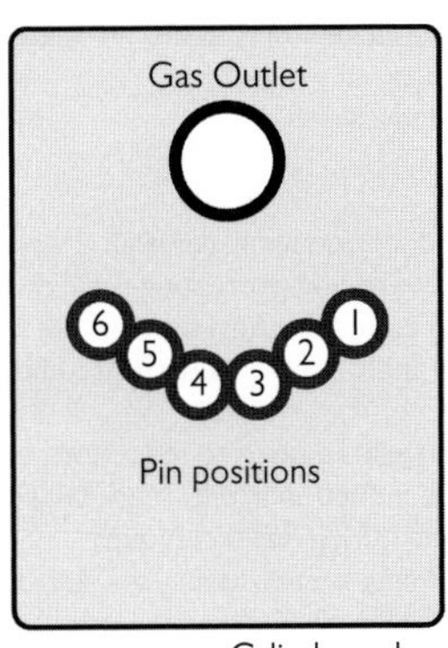

Fig 8.2 An illustration demonstrating the position of pins used in the Pin Index System.

Pitot tube

A pitot tube is a device used to measure a pressure drop as a fluid flows across a fixed resistance. This pressure difference can be used to calculate flow velocity.

In anaesthetic practice, the pitot tube is used to measure tidal volume. The French engineer Henri Pitot described the device in the 18th century.

Index: see Section 1.4.6: Airway pressure; see Section 7.3: Loss of capnography waveform

Preoxygenation

Preoxygenation is an important step in the preparation of a patient for anaesthesia. It requires the breathing of 100% oxygen for around 3 min. This washes out nitrogen from the lungs, replacing it with oxygen.

After an interruption to ventilation, e.g. at induction of anaesthesia, proper preoxygenation can delay a fall in oxygen saturation by several minutes, allowing time for airway manoeuvres to be performed.

Index: see Section 3.4: Planning a general anaesthetic; see Chapter 4: Routine induction of general anaesthesia; see Chapter 5: The rapid sequence induction; see Section 7.2: Airway problems at induction; see Section 7.5: Airway problems at extubation

Related glossary terms: Rapid sequence induction

Propofol

Propofol is a widely used agent for induction and maintenance of general anaesthesia, and for conscious sedation.

At induction, it is generally given at a dose of 2 mg/kg. For TIVA techniques, it is usually given by continuous infusion, often combined with remifentanil.

Propofol can cause pain on injection but causes rapid onset of anaesthesia. Propofol suppresses airway reflexes to a greater degree than other agents, which may facilitate laryngeal mask insertion.

After a single dose, the drug redistributes quickly, so, although propofol has a half-life of 13 h, the patient would be expected to wake in 5–10 min.

Index: see Section 2.2.1: Propofol; see Section 3.4: Planning a general anaesthetic; see Chapter 4: Routine induction of general anaesthesia; see Chapter 5: The rapid sequence induction; see Section 7.5.3: Laryngospasm

Related glossary terms: Remifentanil; TIVA

Racemic mixture

A racemic mixture is one in which both enantiomers of an isomeric drug are present in equal proportions. Bupivacaine is a racemic mixture, as are atropine and many volatile agents.

Index: see Section 2.8: Local anaesthetics

Related glossary terms: Bupivacaine; Enantiomers

Rapid sequence induction

The RSI technique is a method of inducing general anaesthesia to minimize the interval between the patient being fully awake and protecting their own airway to being fully anaesthetized with an airway secured by a cuffed tracheal tube, in the shortest duration possible. Drugs are chosen to be of rapid onset and of short duration so the patient can be awakened in the event of airway problems.

Patients should be fully preoxygenated prior to induction, as the muscle relaxant is traditionally given simultaneously with the induction agent. Mask ventilation is not conducted, so there is higher risk from failed intubation during RSI techniques.

Index: see Section 2.2: Intravenous anaesthetic agents; see Section 2.4.1.2: Rocuronium; see Section 2.4.2.1: Suxamethonium; see Chapter 3: Planning for general anaesthesia; see Chapter 5: The rapid sequence induction; see Section 7.2.4: Difficult intubation during rapid sequence induction

Related glossary terms: Preoxygenation; Sodium thiopental; Suxamethonium

Rebreathing

Rebreathing describes inspiration of a gas mixture that contains CO_2. It is seldom desirable.

Rebreathing is a potential feature when using a Mapleson system with inadequate FGFs, or when using a circle system with an exhausted soda lime canister.

Index: see Section 1.2.9: Breathing circuits

Related glossary terms: Circle breathing system; Fresh gas flow; Mapleson classification; Non-rebreathing circuit; Soda lime

Remifentanil

Remifentanil is a synthetic opioid with potent effects at μ receptors. It has a uniquely short duration of action, and the body's metabolic capacity is very large, so plasma levels do not accumulate even after prolonged infusions.

Although the short duration of action precludes the general use of remifentanil as an analgesic, it is a useful component of many TIVA techniques when administered by target-controlled infusion (TCI).

Index: see Section 3.4: Planning a general anaesthetic

Related glossary terms: Opioid; Opioid receptors; TIVA

Rescue analgesia

Rescue analgesia, also referred to as rescue morphine (or fentanyl) or protocol morphine (or fentanyl), refers to the prescribing of strong opioids on an 'as-required' basis for post-operative patients in the recovery room.

Each recovery area will have its own protocol for the administration of drugs, but generally these involve the administration of set boluses of opioid at given intervals, up to a maximum specified by the anaesthetist (usually 10 mg of morphine or 50–100 micrograms of fentanyl).

It is not appropriate to prescribe rescue doses like this outside of the recovery area. Patients should have their ongoing analgesic requirements met by PCA or via the oral route if strong opioids are required on a continuing basis.

Index: see Section 3.4.4: Post-operative care

Rocuronium

Rocuronium is a non-depolarizing muscle relaxant that acts at nicotinic acetylcholine receptors. It is usually given at doses of 0.6 mg/kg. At lower doses it has a slower onset, comparable to atracurium and vecuronium. It can also be given at higher doses (1.2 mg/kg), at which point the onset time falls to around 60 s. High-dose rocuronium can sometimes therefore be used as a substitute to suxamethonium in cases where suxamethonium would be contraindicated. The duration of action of high-dose rocuronium is around 1 h, so routine use in theatre-based RSI would be discouraged, as it becomes more difficult to manage a failed intubation.

Rocuronium can be reversed using neostigmine and glycopyrrolate, in the same manner as atracurium, but can also be reversed from full relaxation using sugammadex.

Index: see Section 2.4.1.2: Rocuronium; see Chapter 5: The rapid sequence induction; see Section 7.2: Airway problems at induction

Related glossary terms: Neostigmine and glycopyrrolate; Non-depolarizing muscle relaxant; Sugammadex; Suxamethonium

Schrader valve

The Schrader valve is a design of push-to-fit valve for leak-free gas connections. Systems used in the operating theatre are designed with gas-specific collars around the valve pin to prevent misconnection of hoses.

Index: see Section 1.2.1: Piped medical gases; see Section 7.2: Airway problems at induction

Second gas effect

The second gas effect is a useful effect seen when using high concentrations of nitrous oxide. Nitrous oxide is more soluble in blood than volatile anaesthetics and is therefore absorbed from the alveolar space more quickly. Nitrous oxide leaving the gas mixture in the alveolus therefore causes the relative concentration of the remaining anaesthetic agent to rise, setting up a steeper concentration gradient and therefore also speeding its uptake.

The clinical effect is to speed up inhalational induction when nitrous oxide is used in combination with another agent such as sevoflurane.

Index: see Section 2.3: Inhalational anaesthetic agents; see Section 2.3.4: Nitrous oxide
Related glossary terms: Inhalational induction

Sevoflurane

Sevoflurane is an inhalational anaesthetic agent with quick onset and offset. It is useful during inhalational induction of anaesthesia, as it is non-irritant and sweet-smelling. See Table 8.5 for its properties.

Index: see Section 1.2.6: Anaesthetic vaporizers; see Section 2.3: Inhalational anaesthetic agents; see Section 3.4: Planning a general anaesthetic; see Section 7.4: High airway pressures
Related glossary terms: Anaesthetic agent potency; Anaesthetic agent solubility

SI unit

The International System of Units, or SI (taken from the French *Système international d'unités*), is an internationally standardized set of metric units. The system is based on seven fundamental units from which all other units are derived. The fundamental units are given in Table 8.6:

Index: see Section 1.2.3: Pressure gauges
Related glossary terms: Pascal

'Sniffing the morning air' position

This describes the position in which the neck is flexed with the atlanto-axial joint extended. This aligns the upper airway planes and should provide the optimal position for direct laryngoscopy.

Morbidly obese patients may require this position to be modified with the addition of ramping, by which the shoulders are supported with pillows to bring the tragus level with the angle of the sternum.

Index: see Section 7.2: Airway problems at induction

Soda lime

Soda lime is a mixture of sodium and calcium hydroxide, mixed with a pH indicator. The material is formed into granules and stored in a canister mounted in a circle breathing system. As expiratory gas is passed through the canister, the CO_2 reacts with the sodium hydroxide to yield water and sodium carbonate. The calcium hydroxide then reacts with the sodium carbonate to regenerate the sodium hydroxide. The reactions are exothermic so contribute to warming and humidifying the respiratory gas.

Table 8.5 Properties of sevoflurane

	Colour code	MAC	Boiling point	Molecular weight	Blood:gas partition coefficient
Sevoflurane	**Yellow**	**2.00**	**58.5°C**	**200.1**	**0.70**
Isoflurane	Purple	1.10	48.5°C	184.5	1.40
Desflurane	Blue	6.35	22.8°C	168.0	0.45

Table 8.6 Fundamental SI units

Unit	Quantity	Symbol	Unit definition
Mass	Kilogram	kg	1 kilogram is defined by the international prototype kilogram (a platinum–iridium mass stored by the International Bureau of Weights and Measures in Sèvres, France)
Length	Metre	m	1 metre is the distance travelled by light in a vacuum in 1/299 792 458 of a second
Time	Second	s	1 second is the duration of 9 192 631 770 periods of the radiation corresponding to the transition between the two hyperfine levels of the ground state of the caesium 133 atom
Current	Ampere	A	1 ampere is the current which, if maintained in two straight, parallel conductors of infinite length, placed 1 metre apart in a vacuum, would produce a force of 2×10^{-7} newtons per metre of length
Luminosity	Candela	cd	1 candela is the luminous intensity of a source that emits monochromatic radiation (at a frequency of 540×10^{12} Hz) that has a radiant intensity of 1/683 watts per steradian
Amount	Mole	mol	1 mole is the number of elementary particles contained in 0.012 kg of carbon-12
Temperature	Kelvin	K	1 kelvin is 1/273.16 of the thermodynamic triple point of water

As the calcium hydroxide is depleted, the pH rises, reflected in a colour change of the indicator, usually from purple to white, which highlights when the canister needs to be refilled.

Index: see Section 1.2.9.2: Circle systems; see Section 7.3: Loss of capnography waveform

Related glossary terms: Circle breathing system; Rebreathing

Sodium thiopental

Sodium thiopental (also known as sodium thiopentone, thiopentone, or simply 'thio') is a potent thiobarbiturate used for induction of general anaesthesia.

It is most commonly used in RSI, as it is rapid-acting and predictable. An appropriate dose range is 3–7 mg/kg.

Although harmful to tissues if the drug extravasates, it is non-irritant on IV injection. Thiopental produces profound falls in intracranial and intraocular pressures, which may make it of value in the head-injured patient.

The drug is a myocardial depressant and vasodilator so can cause significant falls in blood pressure at induction, particularly in hypovolaemic patients. Care must be taken to volume-resuscitate prior to induction.

Thiopental is rarely given by infusion; the drug accumulates, as the hepatic enzymes responsible for metabolism are easily saturated and levels rise rapidly.

It is contraindicated in patients with porphyria.

Index: see Section 2.2.2: Sodium thiopental; see Section 3.4: Planning a general anaesthetic; see Chapter 5: The rapid sequence induction

Related glossary terms: Rapid sequence induction

Spinal anaesthesia

Spinal anaesthesia involves the placements of a dose of LA into the subarachnoid space. A spinal anaesthetic is typically placed at either L3/4 or L4/5, using narrow-gauge needles with relatively blunt tips to minimize the risk of PDPH.

The most commonly used drug is heavy bupivacaine, a mixture of bupivacaine and glucose, which spreads predictably through the CSF. An opioid, such as fentanyl or bupivacaine, is often added to the mixture.

Spinal anaesthetics usually take around 10 min to develop and last for up to 3 h. They are associated with profound and dense sensory loss in all modalities and loss of motor function. Disruption of sympathetic supply causes vasodilation and hypotension.

Index: see Chapter 6: Central neuraxial blockade

Related glossary terms: Bupivacaine; Heavy bupivacaine

Sugammadex

Sugammadex is indicated for the reversal of neuromuscular blockade resulting from either vecuronium or rocuronium. Unlike neostigmine and glycopyrrolate that can only reverse partial blockade, sugammadex can reverse complete relaxation. Sugammadex is given in doses of 16 mg/kg for emergency reversal.

The drug is relatively expensive, and many hospitals currently reserve its use for emergencies.

Index: see Section 2.4.3.2: Sugammadex

Related glossary terms: Neostigmine and glycopyrrolate; Rocuronium; Vecuronium

Suxamethonium

Suxamethonium is a depolarizing muscle relaxant, commonly used during RSI techniques. It is given in a dose of 1.5 mg/kg and produces muscle relaxation in 30–40 s, with a duration of action of 5–10 min in most patients.

In smaller doses (0.25 mg/kg), it has a role in emergency treatment of laryngospasm. Suxamethonium use is associated with hyperkalaemia, bradycardia, increased ICP, and post-operative myalgia. It is a potential trigger of MH.

Suxamethonium is metabolized by plasma cholinesterase and is prolonged in people with genetic defects in enzyme activity.

Index: see Section 2.4.2.1: Suxamethonium; see Section 3.4: Planning a general anaesthetic; see Chapter 5: The rapid sequence induction; see Section 7.5.3: Laryngospasm

Related glossary terms: Depolarizing muscle relaxant; Laryngospasm; Malignant hyperthermia; Rapid sequence induction; Suxamethonium apnoea

Suxamethonium apnoea

Suxamethonium apnoea describes a genetic abnormality in plasma cholinesterase activity that delays the metabolism of suxamethonium, resulting in prolongation of the drug's action.

Four alleles are recognized (normal, atypical, silent, and fluoride-resistant). Up to one in 25 people may be heterozygotes, in which there is mild prolongation of the effects of suxamethonium of up to 10 min.

In patients who are homozygous for one of the abnormal forms of the enzyme, suxamethonium could be expected to last for 2 h or more.

Index: see Section 2.4.2.1: Suxamethonium; see Section 3.2.1: The anaesthetic history; see Section 7.6: Suxamethonium apneoa

Related glossary terms: Suxamethonium

Tachyphylaxis

Tachyphylaxis describes a decreasing response to a drug with repeated doses. It can occur due to depletion of the neurotransmitters that generate the drug's clinical response (as is the case with ephedrine) or by depletion of the receptors available for mediating its action.

Index: see Section 2.5.1.1: Ephedrine

Related glossary terms: Ephedrine

Tidal volume

Tidal volume, denoted by V_t, is the volume of gas displaced during normal respiratory effort. It is normally approximately 7 mL/kg or around 500 mL in an average-sized adult. The tidal volume is not the same as the volume of gas available for gas exchange (V_A, or alveolar gas volume), as the tidal volume includes dead space.
Index: see Section 1.2.10: The ventilator; see Section 1.4.6: Airway pressure
Related glossary terms: Dead space; Minute volume

TIVA

TIVA is a means of maintaining anaesthesia without the use of an inhaled agent. Although theoretically almost any hypnotic agent could be used, in practical terms propofol is always used to maintain anaesthesia, with or without opioids such as remifentanil.

Modern TIVA techniques use specialized infusion pumps capable of TCI. The anaesthetist programmes the TCI pump with patient details, including height, weight, age, and gender, and then selects a desired plasma or effect–site drug concentration. The pump then uses mathematical models to determine the appropriate infusion rate to reach this concentration.
Index: see Section 1.5: Machine checks; see Section 2.2.1: Propofol; see Section 3.4: Planning a general anaesthetic
Related glossary terms: Remifentanil

Tug-test

This is a test to ensure that pipeline connections to a Schrader valve are secure. The pipeline is given a firm pull to ensure that the valve does not come free and that there are no audible leaks when the traction is applied.
Index: see Section 1.5: Machine checks
Related glossary terms: Schrader valve

Valsalva manoeuvre

The Valsalva manoeuvre consists of forced expiration against a closed glottis. The same effect can be achieved on a ventilated patient by closing the APL valve to maintain a constant positive pressure in the airway.

The manoeuvre has significant cardiovascular effects by raising intrathoracic pressure. The effects are complex but can eventually cause bradycardia. In patients with autonomic dysfunction, it can cause syncope.

Antonio Maria Valsalva originally described the manoeuvre in the 17th century as a means of clearing the Eustachian tube.
Index: see Section 7.10.1: Tachycardia
Related glossary terms: APL valve; Carotid sinus massage

Vasopressor

A vasopressor is a drug that raises systemic vascular resistance to raise blood pressure. Vasopressive drugs are most commonly α-adrenoceptor agonists, although many also possess β-agonist activities too.

Drugs include ephedrine, metaraminol, phenylephrine, and noradrenaline.
Index: see Section 2.5.1.1: Ephedrine; see Section 2.5.1.2: Metaraminol; see Section 2.5.1.3: Adrenaline; see Section 3.4: Planning a general anaesthetic
Related glossary terms: Ephedrine; Inotrope; Metaraminol

Vecuronium

Vecuronium is a non-depolarizing muscle relaxant related to rocuronium. It is a relatively 'clean' drug, with few side effects or significant interactions. Vecuronium is given in doses of

0.1 mg/kg and will yield intubating conditions in 2–3 min. It has a medium duration of action and can be reversed by neostigmine and glycopyrrolate, and by sugammadex.
Index: see Section 2.4.1.3: Vecuronium
Related glossary terms: Neostigmine and glycopyrrolate; Non-depolarizing muscle relaxant; Sugammadex

Vomiting centre

The vomiting centre is a structure in the CNS that receives input from the CTZ, vestibulocochlear system, and directly from the GI tract. The gag reflex, mediated by cranial nerve X, also stimulates the vomiting centre.

The vomiting centre stimulates vomiting by signalling via cranial nerves V, VII, and X.
Index: see Section 2.7: Antiemetics
Related glossary terms: Chemoreceptor trigger zone

WHO analgesic ladder

The WHO analgesic ladder is a suggested approach to analgesic prescribing, first published by WHO in relation to prescribing in cancer. It suggests starting with simple analgesics and gradually introducing more potent drugs in a stepwise manner until pain is controlled.
Index: see Section 2.6: Analgesics; see Section 3.4.4: Post-operative care
Related glossary terms: Codeine phosphate; Diclofenac; Ibuprofen; Morphine sulfate; Non-steroidal anti-inflammatory drugs; Opioid; Paracetamol

Yankauer sucker

The Yankauer suction tip is an oral suctioning device widely used in anaesthetic practice. It is designed to be atraumatic and has a wide tip to accommodate high flow rates.

It is frequently used to suction the oropharynx before and after airway manipulation, and functional suction equipment must be available on every anaesthetic machine.

Charles Yankauer developed the instrument in 1907.
Index: see Chapter 5: The rapid sequence induction

Answers to self-assessment questions

Chapter 1

1. TFTTF—The pin-index system governs the connection of gas cylinders to the anaesthetic machine. The APL valve is a feature of breathing circuits to control the pressure within the system. NISTs manage hose connections at the anaesthetic machine. Schrader valves are hose connections designed to prevent misconnection of gas supplies at the wall. A Bodok seal is a rubber washer that ensures a gas-tight connection between the cylinder and anaesthetic machine.

2. FTFTT—13 700 kPa represents the pressure of a full oxygen cylinder, while 400 kPa is the supply pressure of the oxygen pipeline. Approximate atmopheric pressure can be represented by 1 bar, 762 mmHg, and 101 kPa.

3. FTFFF—A cuffed tracheal tube is the only device that can protect the respiratory tract from soiling after the patient is anaesthetized. An LMA does not form a tight seal over the airway so, although it has a role in rescuing difficult airways, it would not be appropriate as a first choice.

4. TFFFT—Oxygen is carried in white hoses; medical air is carried in black hoses, nitrous oxide in French blue. Oxygen cylinders are black with white shoulders, while air cylinders are grey with black and white shoulders. A nitrous oxide cylinder is blue and contains both liquid and gaseous nitrous oxide. Nitrous oxide is supplied as a piped medical gas in theatre.

5. TFFFF—The SI unit of pressure is the pascal. This is a very small unit of pressure, defined as the force exerted by a 1 kg mass spread over 1 m^2, so more commonly the kilopascal is used. The other units of pressure, although not SI units, are frequently encountered in clinical practice. 1 atmosphere = 1 bar = 101.3 kPa = 1020 cmH_2O.

6. TTTTF—A MacIntosh is the most commonly used laryngoscope blade in adults. A McCoy blade is a modification of the MacIntosh, with a hinge at the end activated by a lever in the handle, while a Polio blade is the same shape as a MacIntosh, but it is mounted on the handle at a different angle. A Magill blade is straight and is generally used in small children.

7. TFFTF—The Mapleson C system is composed of an APL valve, a standard 22 mm connection for the airway, and a reservoir bag. The FGF is connected close to the patient's airway, making it functionally similar to the Mapleson D system. The bag is not self-inflating, so the system must be connected to a gas supply before it can be used. Unidirectional valves and soda lime canisters are features of the circle system.

8. FTFFF—The illustrated circuit is a circle system. The Mapleson system classifies breathing circuits in which there is the possibility of rebreathing at inadequate gas flows, which does not include circle systems. Rebreathing is prevented in a circle by the reaction between soda lime and CO_2. A circle is not suitable for use in small children, because the valves add to work of breathing. This increase is trivial to an adult but could be highly significant in small children. A circle system recycles gas and therefore is highly efficient. It is possible to use gas flows below the patient's minute volume, but it is crucial to monitor the gas composition at the patient's airway; recycling the gases dilutes the FGF, meaning that the concentrations at the patient end do not match the settings on the flowmeter and vaporizer.

9. FFFTT—the Mapleson D system requires 2–4 times the patient's minute volume to adequately wash out expired CO_2 and prevent rebreathing. Mechanical ventilators, such as the Penlon Nuffield 200, can be connected to the bag-mount of a Mapleson D circuit. A Bain circuit is a coaxial Mapleson D circuit. Inspiratory gases are carried from the machine along the inner hose, while expired gases are carried away from the patient along the outer hose.

10. TTFTT—The capnograph waveform gives a lot of information about the patient's respiratory function and airway. During inspiration (A), the waveform should return to 0 (i.e. by point C). If it does not, it implies that the FGF is inadequate (in a Mapleson system) or the soda lime canister is exhausted (in a circle system). Phase B represents expiration as CO_2, exhaled by the patient is detected by the monitor. The end of the expiratory phase (D) gives information about the adequacy of ventilation, while the shape of the upslope of the waveform (E) can change in pathological states such as asthma.

Chapter 2

1. FFFTT—Isoflurane is not suitable for inhalational inductions, as it is a respiratory irritant when awake or lightly anaesthetized. Ephedrine is a sympathomimetic, and atracurium is a non-depolarizing muscle relaxant. Sodium thiopental is a potent barbiturate and classically is used in the RSI. Sevoflurane is a good inhalational induction agent.

2. TTFTF—Propofol does cause vasodilation, and there is some evidence to suggest antiemetic properties. Propofol does not damage tissues if it extravasates, but it does cause pain on injection. Propofol does not provide analgesia.

3. FTTFT—Sodium thiopental is supplied as a powder containing 500 mg thiopental and is usually reconstituted in 20 mL of water for injections. Doses of 3–7 mg/kg are appropriate, but it accumulates when given by infusion as the enzymes responsible for metabolism are easily saturated. Thiopental does reduce ICP. It can trigger acute porphyric crises so is inappropriate for patients with porphyria.

4. FTTTF—Sodium thiopental is not used for maintenance of anaesthesia, as it rapidly accumulates with continuous infusions. It is occasionally given by continuous infusion in ICU practice. Propofol can be given by continuous infusion and is routinely used as part of TIVA techniques. Desflurane and sevoflurane are both inhalational

agents appropriate for maintenance. Midazolam, although suitable for the maintenance of conscious sedation, cannot be used as a sole anaesthetic agent.

5. FTTFT—The MAC of desflurane is 6.35%. The MAC of sevoflurane is 2.00%. The MAC of isoflurane is 1.10%. MAC is not defined in terms of consciousness. It relates to the potency of the agent, representing a concentration of the agent that will prevent movement in response to a standard incision. The MAC of nitrous oxide is theoretically 110%. Although it is a weak anaesthetic agent, its effects are additive with other agents.

6. TFFTF—The sevoflurane vaporizer is colour-coded yellow. Desflurane is presented in a blue vaporizer, and the isoflurane vaporizer is purple. Oxygen and nitrous oxide are not supplied via vaporizer and come instead from piped medical gases or cylinders. The older agents halothane and enflurane were presented in red and orange vaporizers, respectively.

7. FTFFT—Suxamethonium is the only IV agent that triggers MH. All inhalational agents are potentially MH triggers. Non-depolarizing muscle relaxants, propofol, and sodium thiopental are all safe in MH-susceptible patients.

8. FTFFF—Neostigmine and glycopyrrolate are used for the reversal of partial neuromuscular blockade from non-depolarizing muscle relaxants such as atracurium or rocuronium. It cannot be used to reverse suxamethonium. Although mivacurium is a non-depolarizing agent, it has an unusual metabolic pathway and is broken down by the same enzymes as suxamethonium, making it unsuitable for reversal with neostigmine.

9. FTTFT—Ephedrine has mixed α- and β-effects. Stimulation of β_1 receptors causes tachycardia and increased contractility. Glycopyrrolate and cyclizine have anticholinergic effects and therefore raise heart rate. Reflex bradycardias are often seen with drugs that are primarily vasoconstrictors, including metaraminol. Propofol tends to cause bradycardia, especially in children.

10. TFFFT—Morphine is a naturally occurring opioid, derived from the latex of *Papaver somniferum* poppies, with agonist effects at μ, κ, and δ receptors. Low-strength oral morphine solutions are not controlled drugs, although stronger mixtures are. Morphine is not particularly lipid-soluble, so fentanyl or diamorphine are better choices for subcutaneous use. An oral dose of morphine at 20 mg is roughly equal to a 10 mg dose administered IV.

Chapter 3

1. FFTTT—An ASA 1 patient is fit and well, with no other medical conditions. Well-controlled asthma would merit ASA grade 2, although allergy status is not a factor in determining ASA grade. ASA 4 patients have a significant illness that limits day-to-day life. ASA 5 patients are the most unwell and are considered unlikely to survive without surgery.

2. TFFTF—Mallampati II implies incomplete views of tonsils and uvula, but a full view of hard and soft palate. Mallampati grade IV is a predictor of difficult laryngoscopy,

so this patient would not be suitable for an RSI by an inexperienced anaesthetist without careful discussion and assistance from a colleague. The thyromental distance is measured with the neck in maximal extension. Distances <6.5 cm indicate potential difficulties with laryngoscopy. Edentulous and bearded patients may be difficult to mask-ventilate but are not necessarily difficult to intubate.

3. FFFFF—No investigations are required for this ASA 1 patient undergoing this degree of surgery.
4. TFFFT—This patient is fasted, and there are no features to suggest reflux disease, so a routine induction with an LMA would be most suitable, but it would be possible to conduct the case by holding a face mask onto the airway. Tracheal intubation has a greater risk of airway trauma so should only be performed where there is an indication.
5. TTTTF—Any agent could be used to maintain anaesthesia for this type of case, depending on the preference of the patient and the anaesthetist, but all patients require an oxygen-enriched gas supply. Oxygen–nitrous oxide gas mixtures are perhaps less frequently used than oxygen–air, as nitrous oxide use can be associated with post-operative nausea; however, it remains a viable option. Air-only techniques are not suitable.
6. TFTTF—Prescribing post-operatively generally follows the WHO analgesic ladder. The patient has no obvious contraindications to NSAIDs, and regular strong opioids would not generally be required after intermediate surgery such as this. It may, however, be appropriate to prescribe IV fentanyl or morphine as 'rescue' analgesia for use in the recovery room.
7. TTTFF—Coagulation would only be required if there were a suggestion from the history of a bleeding tendency. A chest X-ray would require a specific indication of respiratory pathology.
8. FFFTF—This patient requires an RSI and tracheal intubation. Even if he has not eaten within the last 6 h, the presence of bowel obstruction means he still could not be considered fasted.
9. TTTFF—Any combination of oxygen and either air or nitrous oxide plus one of the volatile agents (isoflurane, sevoflurane, or desflurane) would be appropriate. Nitrous oxide may offer some benefits in this case by allowing the anaesthetist to reduce the amount of volatile required to keep him adequately anaesthetized and therefore minimizing the cardiovascular effects of the anaesthetic. A TIVA technique is very difficult to use when an RSI is required.
10. TTFTF—This patient is undergoing a laparotomy, and significant pain would be expected post-operatively. He will therefore need ongoing strong opioids, but his GI tract will be unreliable in the immediate post-operative phase, meaning that oral morphine may not be effective. As morphine is not particularly lipid-soluble, IM morphine can be unpredictable. An IV PCA is the most practical and convenient means of meeting his opioid needs. If it is possible to give him oral (or IV) paracetamol, with or without an NSAID, it will reduce his overall opioid requirement.

In order to minimize the risk of respiratory depression, it is best not to mix opioids by different routes, e.g. oral codeine with IV morphine.

Chapter 4

1. TFFFF—The recommended dose of propofol is 2 mg/kg, so the most appropriate induction dose would be 140 mg. Although younger patients generally tolerate the drop in blood pressure associated with higher doses well, older patients are more sensitive to the depressant effects of the drugs. Thiopental and suxamethonium are generally reserved for RSIs. Glycopyrrolate would not be routinely drawn up for adult cases, unless there were particular concerns about a risk of bradycardia.
2. TTTTT—All of these factors are checked during the sign-in. The patient will also confirm their identity, that the surgeon has discussed the procedure, and that the surgical site is marked. Patients will be asked if they have metal implants or jewellery, so precautions can be taken to reduce risk of burns associated with diathermy.
3. FFTFT—There are several risk factors associated with PONV. A past history is one, as is being female, a non-smoker, and having a likelihood of requiring post-operative opioids. This patient has two risk factors, so prophylaxis at induction would be indicated. Dexamethasone is probably the most commonly given antiemetic at induction but should not be given while the patient is still awake, as it can cause abnormal perineal sensations. Post-operative use of ondansetron would be appropriate.
4. FFTFF—If a coinduction agent is desired, it should only be given after WHO checks have been completed and monitoring has been established. It should generally be given a few minutes before the induction agent to give it time to take effect.
5. TTTFT—NIBP measured at least every 5 min, continuous ECG, continuous pulse oximetry, and continuous airway gas analysis all form part of minimum monitoring standards set by the AAGBI. Temperature measurement should be made prior to induction of anaesthesia. Peripheral nerve stimulators are mandatory in all cases where a patient has had a muscle relaxant, but continuous use is not required, and monitoring does not need to be started before induction.
6. FFTFT—The recommended dose of vecuronium is 0.1 mg/kg; therefore, this is an appropriate choice. 50 mg atracurium and 100 mg rocuronium would represent an overdosage (atracurium dose is 0.5 mg/kg; rocuronium is normally 0.6 mg/kg—this can rise to 1.2 mg/kg for RSI use). Although the suxamethonium dose is weight-appropriate (1.5 mg/kg), the use of suxamethonium is associated with significant side effects, so it should only be used where there is a specific indication.
7. TFTTT—Capnography is the most reliable method of determining tracheal tube position and must always be checked. Auscultation is important and should be conducted in the mid-axillary line, as transmitted upper airway sounds can be misleading when listening in the mid-clavicular line. Auscultation over the stomach will assist in the detection of oesophageal intubation; in the event of an oesophageal intubation, you will hear abnormal gurgling sounds.

8. FTTFF—This represents a drop in MAP of >50%, so treatment would be required. Metaraminol or ephedrine are both reasonable choices, but metaraminol is typically given in doses of 0.5–1 mg. Glycopyrrolate will raise blood pressure through anticholinergic effects but will tend to raise heart rate to a greater degree, so it would only be indicated if the heart rate were particularly slow. Fluids should be given, as most patients will be volume-deplete when they arrive in theatre.

9. FTFFT—Flow rates need to be reasonably high when first connecting to a circle system to ensure that the hoses are flushed with fresh gas. Tidal volumes should not exceed approximately 7 mL/kg. Once connected, ventilator settings can be titrated to maintain normal E_tCO_2 values and airway pressures of <30 cmH_2O. Either isoflurane or sevoflurane can be used for maintenance, but the isoflurane concentration should not be increased too quickly, as this can cause respiratory irritation.

10. FFFFT—Although suxamethonium ampoules are kept in the refrigerator, it takes time to draw the drug into a syringe. A prefilled syringe will be available to ensure that the drug is immediately ready to use in an emergency. This should also be kept refrigerated.

Chapter 5

1. TFFFT—During an RSI, only the induction agent (thiopental 3–7 mg/kg) and a rapid-acting muscle relaxant (suxamethonium 1.5 mg/kg) should be given. Adding fentanyl or midazolam is not recommended, as it may slow the patient waking up in the event of an unexpected airway problem. Although rocuronium can be used for RSI techniques, it would not be the first choice of drug for an inexperienced anaesthetist, as its long duration of action would delay waking up in an emergency.

2. TTFTT—Always position the airway correctly before beginning an RSI. This will ensure the best possible intubating conditions at the first attempt. A third member of staff is required to be able to seek help in the event of an unexpected problem. After cricoid pressure has started, it should not be released, except in an emergency, so the mobility of the anaesthetic assistant is greatly limited in an RSI. If an NG tube is already present, it would be sensible to connect suction and aspirate it, but placing a new NG tube will only increase patient anxiety and discomfort and may even provoke vomiting or aspiration. The assistant should check where the cricoid is located, prior to induction, so that pressure can be applied as the drugs are being given. Always flush IV cannulae, particularly prior to thiopentone administration as it is highly toxic if it extravasates.

3. TFFFF—The patient should be positioned first, as it is more difficult to move the patient and hold the mask on with a good seal after preoxygenation has started. If preoxygenation is interrupted and the mask removed, it should be repeated for a full 3 min. Suction should be switched on before giving any drugs to minimize delays in the event of regurgitation, and the patient should not be mask-ventilated (except in the case of a failed intubation, as per DAS guidelines plan C; see Section 7.2.3.3), as this can inflate the stomach and provoke regurgitation.

4. TTTTT—Suxamethonium use is complicated by a number of side effects, including MH and anaphylaxis. Bradycardia is seen more commonly in children but can occur in adults. It should be used with caution in patients with pre-existing hyperkalaemia or raised ICP, and care must be taken to identify these patients beforehand.
5. TTTFF—Cricoid pressure should only be released on the explicit instructions of the anaesthetist, but it is appropriate to reduce or remove it if it is impeding the laryngoscopy view (which can happen if it is imperfectly applied). The technique must also be released in the event of active vomiting. Although it can protect against passive regurgitation, active vomiting against cricoid pressure can result in oesophageal rupture.
6. FTTTF—500 mg thiopentone made up in a 20 mL volume yields a 2.5% solution (25 mg/mL); therefore, 11 mL will contain 275 mg. It is important to precalculate the dose that will be given, both in terms of mass and the volume that will be used.
7. FFFFT—Coinduction agents should not be routinely used during an RSI, as they can depress the respiratory drive and slow the patient waking in the event of an unexpected airway difficulty. If a dose of fentanyl is required, it is generally best given after the airway has been secured.
8. FFFTT—The long-acting muscle relaxant should not be given until there is evidence that the suxamethonium has worn off. This might be by checking with a peripheral nerve stimulator or it might be after the patient starts to make spontaneous respiratory effort; this would be noticed as irregular notching of the capnograph trace.
9. FFTTT—Any inhalational agent would be appropriate to maintain anaesthesia after RSI. It is technically very difficult to use a TIVA technique where an RSI is required.
10. TTTFT—Tidal volumes would not normally exceed 7 mL/kg, so a tidal volume of around 575 mL would be appropriate. A normal respiratory rate of around 12 is usually appropriate. Settings would then be titrated to achieve the desired airway pressures (typically peak airway pressure <30 cmH_2O) and E_tCO_2. High-concentration desflurane is a respiratory irritant, so, if desflurane is used, it would usually be started at around 6–8%.

Chapter 6

1. FTTFT—The spinal cord in an adult terminates at the level of the L1–2 interspace. Although the meninges continue onto the conus in the sacrum, they contain only CSF and spinal nerve roots, so it is safe to place a spinal anaesthetic at or below L3–4. Heavy bupivacaine is most commonly used, as the increase in density over CSF means it sinks predictably and the spread of the block can be manipulated by altering the patient's position. Morphine is infrequently used in spinal anaesthetics because it is poorly lipid-soluble. This means that it can be associated with late respiratory depression, as the drug persists in the CSF for a longer period than more lipid-soluble agents (e.g. fentanyl). The block should be well developed by 10 min, so, if there has been no numbness by this point, assistance should be sought.

2. FFFTT—Spinal needles in anaesthetic practice are usually small (25–27G) and have pencil-point tips to part, rather than cut, the fibres of the dura. A dural puncture with a large needle is more likely to cause a PDPH. This is an issue if an accidental dural puncture happens when using a Tuohy needle to site an epidural, as these are typically 16–18G.

3. TTFFF—'Spinals' disrupt all sensory, motor, and autonomic supply below the level of the block, causing vasodilation. This can be sudden, particularly as the block first develops, causing significant hypotension. This can be a serious risk to patients with cardiac disease. Spinal anaesthesia can be used successfully for abdominal operations, including Caesarean section, but the block must proceed to around T4–5 to ensure the peritoneum is adequately anaesthetized. Although not particularly common, it can be combined with general anaesthesia for certain procedures.

4. TTFFF—Tuohy needles are usually either 16 or 18G, much larger than spinal needles. They have markings on the outside at centimetre intervals to make it possible to estimate the depth of the epidural space. The catheter should be placed outside of the dura. If it is accidentally placed below, it will function as a spinal catheter and should not be used without the input of a senior anaesthetist. A loss-of-resistance syringe for epidural use is designed to have low friction. A standard IV syringe is not suitable.

5. FTFTF—An epidural can be placed in either lateral or sitting positions, depending on the patient's and anaesthetist's preference, but the trainee should only perform an epidural in awake patients. Consent is always required, although the process may need to be modified to meet the needs of the patient in acute pain. No more than 5 cm of catheter should be inserted into the epidural space. Inserting an epidural catheter too far increases the likelihood of a unilateral block. Drug doses for spinal anaesthetics are much lower than those used in epidurals.

6. TFTTT—Heavy bupivacaine is only used in spinal anaesthesia, but, provided they are free of preservatives and drawn up with suitable filters and a sterile technique, the other drugs are all suitable for epidural use.

7. TTFTF—The umbilicus is innervated by roots supplied from T10. A block above T4 (corresponding to the level of the nipples) will affect the sympathetic supply to the heart so can cause bradycardia. The xiphisternum is innervated by fibres arising from T6. Tingling in the hands means the block must have reached at least T1. Sensations of chest tightness are not usually a sinister sign and generally result from motor blockade of intercostal muscles which are innervated from the thoracic spine.

8. TTFTF—Before beginning surgery, a block is usually tested for temperature and light touch sensation. It is not usual to test for pain or vibration sensation.

9. FTFFF—Patients on low-dose aspirin can receive an epidural, but patients on clopidogrel must stop this drug at least 7 days in advance. LMWH treatment can continue at prophylactic doses, as long as the first dose is not given within the first 4 h after insertion and the epidural is not removed within 12 h of a dose (24 h must

elapse after a treatment dose). The INR only needs to be checked in a patient who has a specific risk factor, e.g. warfarin treatment or bleeding tendency.

10. TTTTT—All are potentially side effects of both spinal and epidural anaesthesia.

Chapter 7

1. TTFTF—It is vital to call for help as soon as possible, as patients can deteriorate very quickly. No more than three attempts should be made to intubate. Additional attempts merely waste time and potentially prolong hypoxia. The priority in a difficult intubation scenario is patient oxygenation, either with a face mask or an LMA. Unless the surgery is immediately lifesaving, aim to wake the patient up.
2. TFFTF—A completely flat capnograph trace is either a sign of disconnection or total obstruction of the airway. Major haemorrhage may cause CO_2 to fall as a result of decreased delivery to the lungs, but it should not be completely absent. If there has never been a capnograph trace, the airway is not in the correct location. In pneumothorax, there should still be detectable CO_2 in the expired gas.
3. FFTTT—Disconnection should cause a fall in airway pressure, while major haemorrhage should have no effect on airway pressure. The others all represent obstructions at various levels of the respiratory system or airway and would therefore cause pressures to rise.
4. TTFFT—The mainstay of treatment in anaphylaxis is IM adrenaline, along with steroids, antihistamines, and bronchodilators. IV adrenaline is occasionally required but should not be administered without great caution. IV fluids are vital, but crystalloids are generally recommended, as colloids can themselves be triggers of anaphylaxis. Chloramphenicol is an antibiotic and has no role in the treatment of anaphylaxis. Treatment with chlorphenamine (an antihistamine) is indicated; the dose is 10–20 mg IV.
5. FFTFF—This rhythm is VF, and cardiac arrest should be suspected. Although VF is not compatible with a cardiac output, motion artefact can give monitor appearances identical to VF, even when the patient still has a pulse. DC cardioversion is not appropriate for a cardiac arrest rhythm. Defibrillation is the definitive management of cardiac arrest secondary to VF. Adrenaline is not required until after the third shock has been delivered.
6. TFTFF—VF should be treated by defibrillation. Adrenaline is indicated after the third shock, along with amiodarone. Neither atropine nor pacing have a role in cardiac arrest, although both may be used in the treatment of a patient with a symptomatic bradycardia.
7. FFTFT—A 1 in 10 000 solution implies 1 g is diluted into 10 000 mL, so 1 mg is contained in 10 mL of a 1 in 10 000 solution, or 1 mL of a 1 in 1000 solution.
8. FTFFF—This rhythm is VT. As the patient has a pulse but shows adverse signs (hypotension, signs of cardiac failure, signs of cardiac ischaemia), synchronized DC cardioversion is appropriate. In the conscious patient, this will generally require

some form of sedation or anaesthesia. Amiodarone may be required if three shocks are unsuccessful, but it would not be first-line management.

9. TFFFT—Carotid sinus management is used in the treatment of patients with no adverse features who present with regular narrow complex tachycardias. Care should be taken with the patient with sinus tachycardia; in anaesthetic practice, this is usually secondary to other causes such as haemorrhage or inadequately deep anaesthesia. Correcting these factors is usually sufficient to control the tachycardia. DC cardioversion should be considered for unstable patients with adverse features.

10. TFFFT—MH is triggered by suxamethonium and inhalational anaesthetics. Hyperthermia is a late sign, and the condition generally presents as an unexplained rise in E_tCO_2, with a tachycardia. Definitive treatment is with dantrolene (intralipid is used for LA toxicity), and patients should be referred to the MH Investigation Unit in Leeds for follow-up. Tryptase is the investigation required after anaphylaxis.

Index

Note: Page numbers in *italics* refer to figures, tables, and boxes.

P

R

S